POSITIVE PARENTING SOLUTIONS TO RAISE HIGHLY SENSITIVE CHILDREN

UNDERSTANDING YOUR CHILD'S EMOTIONS AND HOW TO RESPOND WITH RADICAL COMPASSION, LOVE AND CONFIDENCE

JONATHAN BAURER

Positive Parenting Solutions to Raise Highly Sensitive Children

Understanding Your Child's Emotions and How to Respond with Radical Compassion, Love and Confidence

First Published in 2022

by Exploring Changes

Asheville, North Carolina - USA

https://exploringchanges.com

ISBN paperback: 978-1-958012-01-7
ISBN hardback: 978-1-958012-02-4
ISBN e-book - PDF: 978-1-958012-04-8
ISBN E-book – Epub: 978-1-958012-05-5
ISBN audiobook: 978-1-958012-03-1
Library of Congress Control Number: 2022904747

For more information, please contact:
jon@exploringchanges.com

FIRST EDITION

Let's Connect!

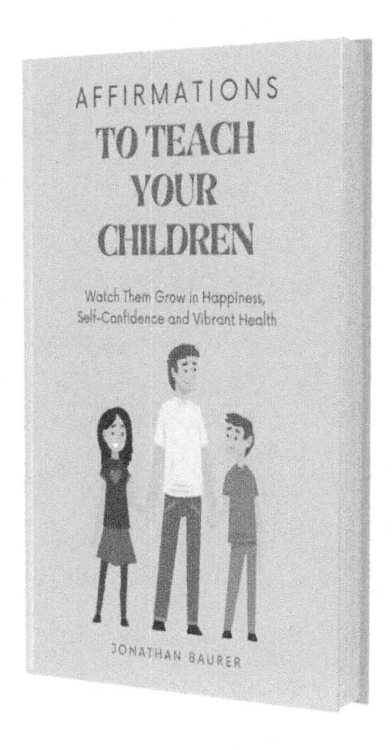

Scan to join my email list to receive a FREE ebook and occasional updates!

CONTENTS

INTRODUCTION

Every child is special and unique, gifting us with abundant memories, joys, and love. They grow and develop their own personalities, curiosities, and views of the world in ways many adults cannot even begin to fathom. Sometimes, their perspective can be magically different from our own, and while every child needs care and love, some just need a bit more understanding, comfort, and empathy.

With sharp and in-depth views of the world, these children are intellectually, creatively, and emotionally gifted, showing mature compassion even in their early years. Highly sensitive children (HSC) have a keen awareness; they are highly empathetic, emotional, and deep thinkers. This high awareness can become over-stimulating; they can become overwhelmed by crowds, sounds, new environments, changes, and the emotional distress of those around them. This type of over-stimulation requires parents and caregivers to be highly empathetic, compassionate, and perceptive.

You might already have a basic understanding of what a highly sensitive child is, or maybe the term is completely new to you. Things that might seem usual or bearable for us can be viewed quite differently by HSC. They might struggle with perfectionism, ask numerous questions to satisfy their abundance of curiosity, become highly affected by others' emotions, or become overwhelmed by noises or surprises. Some HSC might struggle to fall asleep or feel comfortable in certain clothes. These children can also be wary of new experiences, needing the right amount of stability and predictability to help them feel comfortable in new situations.

While there might be numerous triggers unique to each child, one thing is certain: patience, understanding, and positivity are a must when caring for HSC. With the right encouragement and support, these children will grow and thrive in their environments, becoming more resilient over time.

Parenting and/or caring for highly sensitive children can become overwhelming and frustrating. However, if we switch our mindsets to better understand ourselves and these children, we reap extremely rewarding activities and relationships in return. Discovering your own gift through developing specific parenting skills will help you embrace and support your healthy, well-adjusted highly sensitive child.

Being a parent or a caregiver is a unique experience. Through it, we experience journeys of growth and development and help shape the future. Children look to their parents, teachers, and other adults for guidance, support, and safety, and we can provide all these things and more.

Sensitive children need good role models as they learn to use their special gifts in a world that might not always understand them. We will go through a detailed, step-by-step guide on creating and maintaining a positive parenting experience with incredible and beneficial results for raising resilient highly sensitive children. The techniques and strategies you will learn will give you an advantage as you develop your own radical compassion, love, and confidence.

I have been studying positive parenting solutions for 20 years, utilizing my knowledge and research with my own sensitive child. As a life coach, I understand the unique and often stressful challenges that parents and caregivers of highly sensitive children face. My goal is to help you better understand the needs of your HSC, help you gain peace of mind as you navigate this journey toward a positive parenting style, and support awareness of your child's gifts.

My wife is a highly sensitive person, and I am not; but we have both enjoyed amazing and positive experiences using the techniques you will be studying in this book. Our aim is to help others achieve the same outcome. Over time, I have developed an excellent understanding of how a highly sensitive child is wired and how to nurture them using elements of empathy, understanding, and patience. We will dive into and explore these tools together so that you can begin using them today.

Taking these steps now demonstrates your desire and willingness to be proactive. After reading this book, you'll be able to assess your own strengths and weaknesses when it comes to positive parenting, improve your understanding and empathy when caring for a highly sensitive child, and develop a better understanding of yourself.

Let's step into the unique, creative, and beautiful world of a highly sensitive child and create a more fulfilling, connected, and compassionate world together.

CHAPTER 1

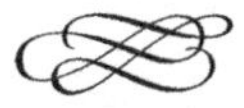

THE SUPER KIDS

If you've picked up this book, you've noticed signs that you may have a highly sensitive child. Perhaps you've seen them fidget with the irritating tags on their clothing or gravitate towards quieter environments. Maybe you've recognized that your child is more perceptive than others their age or that they have an unquenchable thirst for knowledge and understanding of the world around them. Some people might have labeled your child as "highly emotional" or "volatile" simply because they had no understanding or words to describe how uniquely wonderful your kid really is.

Elaine Aron describes highly sensitive children as "one of the 15 to 20 percent of children born with a nervous system that is highly aware and quick to react to everything" (Lodestone Center n.d.). While this term might still be obscure, it has started to pop up more frequently as behavioral health professionals push to help caregivers and parents better understand these overlooked and mislabeled children.

UNDERSTANDING YOUR SPECIAL KID

The first thing to understand about HSC is that these children struggle to deal with stimuli that might seem normal or common to others. These stimuli include lights, sounds, smells, activities, or even other people's emotions, which can easily overwhelm them, especially in crowds. Reactions to over-stimulation can manifest in emotional or behavioral difficulties, but it comes with benefits, as well.

Common positive characteristics of highly sensitive children include creativity, intellectuality, and emotional maturity. HSC are often highly attuned to the emotions of others, making them sympathetic and compassionate individuals. And though you might have experienced some pickiness, sensory difficulties, shyness, or hyperactivity, once understood, I wouldn't call them "negative traits."

In order to understand our HSC, we must change our own thought patterns. Pickiness is not just being finicky but needing familiarity. Being introverted isn't a bad thing; it just means they feel more comfortable on their own than surrounded by others. Hyperactivity is a great thing to have for sports or to pursue other interests.

Society has told us these types of behaviors are not the norm or aren't valuable, but there is value if we look at it in a new light and cast off the social conditioning we've become so used to. We're led to believe that these children do not fit in. However, not conforming isn't a bad thing at all.

While our world believes that these children are deficient in certain areas, as a parent or caregiver of a highly sensitive child, you understand that your child can grow in so many wonderful ways with the right support and guidance. The key? Recognizing that a highly sensitive child needs a highly compassionate parent to understand them.

Let's focus on five traits of highly sensitive children: intense emotional reactions, deep processing of experiences, being highly empathetic toward others, becoming easily overstimulated, and sensitivity to even the most subtle stimuli.

HSC can feel more intense joy and fear, anger and sadness. They might cry easily or have their feelings hurt more often than other children their age. They will be more inclined to contemplate than rush into action and will often be described as withdrawn, timid, or shy. Around 70 percent of highly sensitive people are considered introverts (Wilson n.d.).

Highly sensitive children can become overstimulated easily and then require rest or time to themselves to recharge. Seemingly small or subtle stimuli, which others might not even notice, can be very upsetting to HSC. Simple things—such as itchy fabrics or clothing tags, the weather and temperature, and certain outdoor textures, such as sand or grass—can agitate them, whereas their siblings or peers seem unbothered. Loud or busy environments might cause emotional or physical stress, and they'll be more sensitive to background noises or sounds, such as the clinking of silverware together at a restaurant or utensils scratching against a plate.

Highly sensitive children often show great concern for those around them. They exhibit great empathy and compassion, even towards strangers. They feel eager to please and are concerned about doing things the "right way." HSC often seem mature for their age, asking in-depth and thoughtful questions beyond their years. HSC have the special ability to pick up on subtle social cues just by paying close attention to body language or facial expressions. They often have exceptional intuition.

What we need to understand as parents and caregivers of HSC is that these children view the world differently than we do. They're able to see, feel, and experience things in a different light, and we must try to see the world from their point of view. If we are willing to join them in this experience, our highly sensitive children will teach us a thing or two about love, compassion, patience, and adaptation.

UNDERSTANDING THE BRAIN OF YOUR HIGHLY SENSITIVE CHILD

The term "highly sensitive person" (HSP) was first used by psychologist Dr. Elaine Aron (Lear 2021). She defined HSP as individuals wired in a more sensitive way. They have stronger reactions to everyday stimuli such as strong sounds, odors, or sights that don't normally affect others. They also feel stronger emotions than the average individual.

One thing we need to note before truly understanding the brains of our incredible children is that this is not a mental disorder; it is a personality trait with extra flair. It is not a problem to be solved but a difference to be celebrated. Just as someone can be more extroverted or talkative, some individuals are more sensitive than others.

When it comes to truly understanding highly sensitive children, we should keep a couple Cs in mind: caution and consequences.

Highly sensitive children are cautious, automatically assessing the environment around them. They have a strong "pause-to-check" system that allows them to compare current experiences to past ones and notice similarities. Unfamiliar sensory experiences or a flood of strange stimuli can be overwhelming for highly sensitive people. Taking time for comparison helps them adjust to new situations and adapt, allowing them to process strange environments or circumstances and assist them in feeling more comfortable.

The first C, *caution*, gives highly sensitive children a keen sense of potential *consequences*. Due to their mature processing skills, HSC can imagine and map out the impact of the consequences to their actions in ways neurotypical children can not. It helps them mitigate risks and protect themselves and those around them. However, one of the biggest obstacles for a highly sensitive child is to live life without the fear of each unpleasant possibility, though it is certainly not always the drawback some might think it is. This just means that, as parents or caregivers, we must help our child to alleviate the usual stress that can develop from this type of processing.

Highly sensitive children sometimes struggle with their need for perfection—to do tasks correctly and thoroughly before being able to move on to something else. HSC can be incredibly self-conscious and, where an average individual might accept mistakes as a normal part of being human, highly sensitive people feel that they themselves aren't enough.

Normal activities such as public speaking, recitals, big assessments, assignments, or exams easily stress HSC out, causing them to present less than they're truly capable of. With guidance and support, HSC can learn how to adapt to situations that, without support, can fill them with dread. Accepting their mistakes rather than letting them affect their self-confidence is a critical life skill.

Dr. Elaine Aron was able to define the characteristics of a highly sensitive child, shedding more light on the way these children think and see the world. However, the question still remains—why? Why are highly sensitive children prone to perfectionism and emotional reactivity? Why do normal stimuli tend to stress them out while their peers and siblings remain unbothered?

HOW THEY PROCESS INFORMATION

As mentioned before, high sensitivity doesn't develop over time, and it is not a mental disorder or a problem. Highly sensitive people are just wired differently than others—and that's not a bad thing! It's not even an uncommon thing.

Sensory processing sensitivity is a biological trait roughly represented in about a third of the world's population (Fernandez 2021). Highly sensitive people are viewed as having intense highs and lows, coupled with extreme or erratic caution. These traits are due to the different ways HSP brains process the world around them.

Most research studies have revolved around how the brain reacts to stimuli. One study, conducted by Bianca Acevedo, a psychologist at Santa Barbara's University of California, took this research a step further to understand where this deeper processing takes place in the brain.

Using a functional magnetic resonance imaging scanner, researchers had HSC engage in tasks with different descriptions of emotions, such as happy or sad, followed by the corresponding faces of their partners and strangers. The participants were then asked to count backward to reset between each of the photos (Fernandez 2021).

Acevedo and the other researchers found a pattern that suggested a sensitive person's brain continued to show the activity of deep processing, even during rest. This continued brain activity is a key component of high sensitivity.

WHY YOUR CHILD IS HIGHLY SENSITIVE

As humans, we have two primary response strategies to our environments: think before acting or act before thinking. Our response often depends on our personality traits. However, a highly sensitive child has a third reaction: sensory processing sensitivity (Betancort 2020).

This response allows a highly sensitive person to process the environment around them in a more in-depth way. It allows them to perceive more detail than others, integrating information to better respond.

This trait has been studied not only on a behavioral level but a genetic one, as well. Some studies have found a relationship between the levels of sensitivity and polymorphism of a specific gene called the 5-HTTLPR (Daw et al. 2013). This gene is specifically related to increased sensitivity to one's environment and has also been linked to superior performance in tasks and decision-making. Studies have shown a correlation between the sensory processing sensitivity trait and dopamine. Highly sensitive children do not just see the world differently—they're genetically wired for it.

But what does this mean exactly? A highly sensitive person's brain configuration is linked to their deep but subtle processing of both their environment and emotions. They can identify the moods of those around them and are more aware of individual emotional states, especially positive ones. This research has shown that highly sensitive people tend to process more positive emotions than negative or neutral ones—which, of course, is a great thing!

Being highly sensitive is not a mental disorder or mental problem—it's simply a personality trait. Elain Aron uses an acronym to better define what a highly sensitive person experiences: *DOES.*

D: Depth of Processing

O: Overstimulated

E: Emotional Reactivity/Empathy

S: Sensitivity to Subtle Stimuli

Highly sensitive brains will think more deeply about things they need to do and notice more connections between all of the pieces of information they process. This attention to detail enables them to be more thorough during tasks or projects, more creative, and think outside the box.

However, this attention to detail can cause HSC to become easily stressed or overwhelmed, so they require downtime to recharge, especially after strenuous social activities. However, this isn't always the case. There are actually some HSC who require stimulation, called high sensation seekers (Highly Sensitive Society n.d.). These types of HSC might seek out or adopt thrill-seeking behaviors. They might even develop a fear of missing out—a complete opposite to most HSC.

Still, even high sensation seekers cannot handle overwhelming stimuli for very long and will often bounce between seeking stimulation and recharging.

Though there might be a difference between HSC and stimulation-seeking behaviors, one thing remains the same: they are highly perceptive to the subtle stimuli in their environments. They can perceive stimuli beyond that of an average individual and often have stronger intuitions. Each child is, of course, unique, though they still share the same propensity to elevated levels of sensitivity. Some HSC might be extra intuitive and empathetic, while others might become overwhelmed by physical stimuli.

Surprisingly, this is not just a human personality trait. High sensitivity has been found in over 100 animals, as well. It's considered biological—not just mental. Those who have studied it are discovering correlations between high sensitivity to serotonin and dopamine genes, as well as linking it to specific brain areas.

Highly sensitive children are not highly sensitive due to their environments—they're born with it. And, most likely, someone along their family tree also had the same trait.

IT'S NOT A DIAGNOSIS

When researching highly sensitive children, you might come across something called sensory processing disorder (SPD). It's not uncommon to mistake the two. However, high sensitivity is not a disorder to be diagnosed, as I've stated before, but a genetic personality trait.

SPD is when children find it difficult to combine the information they receive through the senses in a more organized way (Jagiellowicz 2019). This disorder used to be categorized on the autism spectrum but has since been labeled as its own disorder.

Highly sensitive people might appear to have traits that align with SPD, but there is a key difference between the two. A highly sensitive person will not typically experience problems doing everyday activities and can learn to adapt to stressful stimuli, which is not common for children with SPD. In actuality, research has shown that highly sensitive individuals are better at integrating sensory information than those with SPD (Jagiellowicz 2019).

Children who are highly sensitive and those diagnosed with SPD can both be affected by over stimulating events, and some highly sensitive children might also show certain sensory sensitivities (Gere et al. 2009). So how, as a parent or caregiver, do you identify your child's needs?

Research has shown that it's all about how their brains process information differently. Highly sensitive children are not overreacting—they are responding to subtle stimuli that non-highly sensitive individuals tend to miss. The more a highly sensitive person responds, the more their brain is actually paying attention to details.

It's important to remember that there are four facets to HSC and HSP in general. To be labeled highly sensitive, the child must show greater empathy toward others than most children their age, be able to identify and pay attention to the minute details in their surroundings, be detail-oriented in tasks or work, and feel more moved by art, music, or other beautiful details than non-highly sensitive individuals.

Identifying whether or not someone has sensory processing sensitivity (SPS) or is highly sensitive (HS) can be complicated. And while there are tests out there for research purposes, these self-reported assessments shouldn't be treated as the final word on any personality trait, mental disorder, or temperament trait. Many studies have used these tests as a form of measurement—not a diagnosis.

The tests you find online will not be true indicators of your child's sensitivity. The best way for you to determine if your child is highly sensitive is by reading, researching, and developing your own understanding about the traits.

High sensitivity can be found in almost 20 percent of the population, though mistakes in identifying HSC can be made (Aron n.d.). For example, high sensitivity is sometimes mistaken for a disorder. According to the Diagnostic and Statistical Manual of Mental Disorders (DSM-5), a disorder is only present when it causes significant distress or impairment in important functioning, such as social activities or professional work. Of course, distress is subjective, and highly sensitive children or adults will certainly feel distressed when over-stimulated. However, at this time, it is not labeled as a mental disorder, nor should it be treated like one.

You also need to note the common mislabeling of non-highly sensitive persons. Some people believe they are highly sensitive people when they are not, and many parents might jump to assumptions that their child also struggles with this when they are simply being themselves. However, HS can occur alongside other significant challenges, and if a parent or caregiver truly believes there is an issue, they should certainly seek out professional assistance.

If you feel uncertain about what is going on, it is always appropriate to get an opinion from a professional. Going to an expert, especially one who has experience with children or specializes in child psychology, is a great way to better understand what is going on. They will be able to get to know your child and how they react in a variety of situations; they can assess your child's behavior and assist in providing helpful resources.

CHAPTER 2

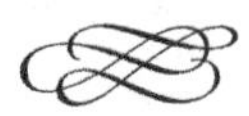

LOOKING THROUGH THEIR EYES

For anyone to truly understand others, we should step into their shoes and see through their eyes. The same could be said for parents and caregivers of highly sensitive children. We must be willing to really get into their heads and try to view the world as they do. This not only helps us better understand our children, but it allows us to understand why they choose to behave or respond the way they do.

There are many different facets to being highly sensitive. Some of these might feel challenging. Yet, the only reason why most would label these certain aspects "challenging" is because they really don't understand them.

Once we understand the world in which highly sensitive people live, we can help our children navigate this life. Many of the characteristics of high sensitivity are easily remedied with just a little more understanding and access to the right tools.

COMMON CHALLENGES FOR HIGHLY SENSITIVE CHILDREN

When it comes to being a highly sensitive child, emotions often run deep and sometimes overflow. HSC may feel overwhelmed or stressed in different areas of their lives. This stress can show up as general anxiety, exhaustion, poor concentration, or even lowered immune function. For HSC, even pleasant experiences can be draining. Here are some other common highly sensitive challenges you might experience with your child:

- They react strongly to both positive and negative experiences.
- They have an abundance of feelings and the ability to tune into the emotions of those around them.
- Large crowds can be intense. HSC usually prefers one-on-one interactions and making meaningful connections rather than being social butterflies.
- Symptoms of anxiety or depression are common, especially when children lack a secure attachment with a significant adult.
- Loneliness can be a challenge when they feel misunderstood or different from family and peers.
- Oftentimes, this feeling of being different comes when a highly sensitive child feels as if they're falling behind. They might believe that they're slower to hit the 'normal' milestones their friends and peers are achieving.

While some non-sensitive individuals might understand these challenges, others may not. Opening our minds and enhancing our own empathy can help us see where HSC are coming from. You do not have to understand what a highly sensitive child feels through first-hand experience, but you can learn about and acknowledge their challenges.

WHAT TRULY MATTERS

While there are many general qualities listed in this book about how a highly sensitive child views the world, in reality, each HSC is unique. Some things matter more to a highly sensitive child—things that make them different from others their age. These differences are not odd or wrong but something to be celebrated and explored.

One highly sensitive child might have an especially heightened sense of smell, whereas another highly sensitive child might be more affected by sounds. One might be able to handle crowds better than another. As parents and caregivers, we need to help our highly sensitive child understand their superpowers so they can cultivate their own sense of identity. Understanding their specific needs will also allow you to aid them in exploring different ways to cope with or regulate these emotions and challenges.

One of the ways you can assist them in regulating their river of feelings is by contemplative practice. Meditation, practicing mindfulness, or any other reflective activity is essential for a highly sensitive child. These types of thoughtful and deeply nurturing practices affirm and support HSC, meeting their needs for assessing their true emotions and learning more about their experiences.

Many HSC will avoid anything that makes them feel discomfort, especially negative feelings. This can create a never-ending cycle, a downward spiral, but it doesn't have to be this way. Avoidance is key to a highly sensitive child when it comes to stressful situations. As parents, we can help them embrace and reconfigure their discomfort in ways that help them maintain their positivity and create space for more positive feelings.

As parents, it is critical that we highlight all of our HSC's sensitive strengths. For example, their love of art, music, and nature, along with their imagination, can all be beneficial coping mechanisms. These interests can also help our children build more resilience as they face the real world.

TRAITS OF A HIGHLY SENSITIVE CHILD

For people who don't know better, when they think of the term "highly sensitive," they might picture someone who cries easily, has thin skin, or is distressed at the slightest provocation. Yet, as parents and caregivers of HSC know, there is more to their temperament than simply feeling too much. Highly sensitive children have hyper-aware nervous systems and react quickly (Drudi n.d.).

In addition to Elaine Aron's DOES acronym, other signs might indicate your child is highly sensitive. HSC are incredibly empathetic. Other people's emotions can be highly triggering for them as they feel these emotions more intensely than non-highly sensitive individuals. Empathy is one of the main facets of high sensitivity.

Highly sensitive children process things very deeply. They tend to think about any and all possibilities, which often presents as probing questions and difficulty making decisions. They pay attention to details in every aspect of their lives, fueling their incredible thirst for understanding and knowledge.

To non-highly sensitive people, the sensitivity of HSC may seem super-powered. They're quick to notice subtle changes in their environment and the people around them. Most people probably hate the sound of nails on a chalkboard or feedback from a microphone, but to a highly sensitive child, even the sound of a fork scraping against a plate or a cardboard box being opened can not only sound too loud and feel over-stimulating, it may actually be painful.

Super senses can bleed into pickiness over clothing. It's not that they prefer their Spiderman shirt to their Iron Man one; it's the textures of the cloth, the material, and even the tags that can be unbearably uncomfortable for HSC. Wet and sand-filled clothing might feel uncomfortable for most people, but for HSC, it's nearly impossible to tolerate.

Highly sensitive children may also find sleeping and new

activities to be a struggle. Due to their active minds and heightened awareness, getting HSC to sleep can be more challenging than with non-highly sensitive children. Drifting off when they have so much to think about can be extremely difficult. This heightened brain activity also means that HSC need time to adjust to new activities; they will need time to prepare and get ready to process all the new stimuli they will encounter.

If your child exhibits most, if not all, of these very specific traits, you might have a highly sensitive child. The behaviors of a highly sensitive child are specific and well-defined, based on research of this personality trait. Parenting a highly sensitive child can be an absolute gift, and you can rise to meet seemingly impossible challenges with understanding and a sensitive approach, which we will cover later in this book.

SHY OR HIGHLY SENSITIVE?

It's not uncommon for highly sensitive people to be labeled as "shy." However, there is a difference between HSP and shy individuals; in fact, roughly 30 percent of highly sensitive individuals are actually extroverts (Eby 2021).

Shyness is partly due to genetics as well as influenced by learned behaviors, though no one is necessarily born shy—unlike HSC, which has been found to be linked to genetics alone. There are many possible causes of shyness, especially in children and young adults.

Children, in general, learn by imitating their parents or caregivers, and children who are isolated from other children may fail to develop the necessary social skills that allow them to interact easily with others. Shyness can develop from various influences in a child's life—but it is not necessarily the same thing as being a highly sensitive child.

If anything, introverts and highly sensitive people might have more behaviors in common than either have with people who are "shy." Due to overstimulation, highly sensitive individuals need to recharge their batteries, much like introverts. They both need a non-stimulating place to give their senses a break.

As parents and caregivers of HSC, it is important to stay away from the possible harmful label of "shyness." HSC can be extroverts or introverts. Both personality types can enjoy social situations as long as they are able to cope with the unique challenges of the stimuli they perceive. We just need to understand their needs.

MAKING SENSE OF THE OUTBURSTS

We've established that highly sensitive children can become easily overwhelmed by their environment and that these children have energy to spare. This feeling of being overwhelmed or distressed can often present itself in the form of anger or frustration.

Anger is a part of being human; it is our natural fighting instinct taking over, a shield we might use to protect ourselves even as adults. Children are no different, and it shouldn't be a cause of concern. There are many ways in which parents and caregivers can help ease and guide this energy into feelings and actions that are positive and adaptable.

Understanding why children feel angry is the first step in helping them. This emotion indicates that something is off-balance and will often hide other emotions or feelings. There are many causes of anger: tiredness, overstimulation, physical distress, hunger, feeling misunderstood or overwhelmed—especially for highly sensitive children.

As parents, we may find our children's energy overwhelming; we may struggle to understand. It can be easy to label this energy as manic or struggle with other diagnoses simply because you aren't aware of how your highly sensitive child's system works.

There are a few key components when it comes to raising HSC—things we need to see in a new light in order to help guide and support them.

The first key piece in this puzzle is to recognize that sensitive children do tend to have more energy than "normal" children, which might sound astounding as children, in general, are known for their endless amounts of liveliness. With HSC, this energy can be intense, and this intensity is what most parents notice when it comes to tantrums or outbursts.

Some sensitive children can shift instantly from happy to sad; others appear stuck or seem to flounder aimlessly through emotional shifts and seemingly unrelated actions. Like other children, they will need to learn how to manage their emotions and direct their thoughts and actions, just as any child does. Learning about this piece of the puzzle helps them to channel their superpower energy effectively.

Once they learn how to channel their emotions and feelings, they can use this energy for great things. Like Jack Andraka, a highly sensitive child who found a break-though for cancer at the age of 15, your child can thrive in their interests rather than constantly battling them. HSC can use their superpowers for amazing things if they can effectively embrace, use, and channel their energy.

SEE THE LIGHT

As I've already begun pointing out, there are incredible benefits to being highly sensitive. As a parent or caregiver, it's easy to see just how amazing our children can be. However, due to their hyper-awareness of their environment and those around them, highly sensitive children will realize that they are, indeed, different and may come to believe that other people view this fact in a negative way.

They might wonder or ask why they can't just be "normal." They might experience negative spirals thinking of all the ways they are different from their friends. Part of your job is to continuously remind them how very special they are!

Most HSC are incredible when it comes to tuning into other people's emotions. Their empathy can rival Mother Teresa's, and their compassion and care for those around them is something to be celebrated. They can easily picture themselves in other people's shoes, making them great listeners and compassionate human beings.

Many HSC are also amazingly creative. They have highly imaginative minds and can view the world differently than most in such a unique way. They are able to bring beauty into the world, even when non-highly sensitive people cannot see it.

Being very detail-oriented, HSC notice many things most non-highly sensitive people do not. They're observant and will often have heightened senses, such as a better sense of touch, smell, taste, or sight.

Noticing these details often leads them to think more in-depth about how the world works around them. They love to question and love to learn. Their thirst for understanding is unquenchable —and that's something we need in this world.

Overall, HSC want to make the world a better place. They understand the hardships of those around them and wish to help those in need.

There are many positive aspects to HSC. While others might view these qualities as too energetic or shy or any number of negative labels, we know how special they really are. And it's *your* job to constantly remind them of that.

PREFERENCES

Highly sensitive children have strong preferences for everything from learning behaviors to their nutritional needs, as well as how they connect to others and the environments they prefer.

It should go without saying that HSC learn differently from non-sensitive people. They learn best through their senses, their bodies, and their spirits. Their imaginative and creative minds make them visual learners who do best in a more holistic education than a step-by-step process.

This type of education concept—focusing on the entirety of

an individual beyond just academics—allows for all of the senses to play a key part in learning. HSC see the world through sensory details, emotional awareness, and heightened empathy—something holistic education is centered around.

One thing to remember when it comes to a highly sensitive child's learning needs is that they must be able to filter the various energies around them to focus. This is especially important to HSC who are still adapting to their sensory systems and cannot understand why they get overwhelmed just yet.

HSC need to be able to move along at their own pace, whether in an educational setting or throughout their daily activities. Many are often seen as perfectionists, though it's more than just that. Due to the way they process information, HSC move a little slower than others. They might need more time to complete different tasks or make decisions.

Due to this detailed way of processing their surroundings, HSC actively avoid anything that might overwhelm or upset them. They tend to dodge confrontation, dramatic discipline, excess noise, and other overwhelming situations. And, after encountering such episodes, they'll often retreat to a safe space.

Many HSP, children included, prefer to have a safe haven where they can recharge after activities. The onslaught of sensory details and overstimulation will make them feel as if they cannot keep up with all these activities. They sometimes prefer intervals of work, rest, and then work again, integrating something they can easily focus on before regrouping.

Their preferred spaces might include low lighting, a place with little noise, and—because they are able to fully appreciate the beauty around them—a nice aesthetic. Their safe haven might also include their favorite things to help them relax, such as books, music, or comfortable pillows to make the space physically and emotionally comfortable.

Like most people, children will have their preferences when it comes to food. With HSC, however, these preferences can often be mislabeled as simply being a "picky eater." Eating food is a sensory experience, including different textures, aromas, temperatures, and tastes. These different stimuli can all affect a highly sensitive child more than others.

For example, HSC can be quite sensitive to certain ingredients, such as caffeine. Caffeine tricks our brain into releasing "feel good" chemicals, such as dopamine and serotonin, in addition to adrenaline and norepinephrine, which are actively involved in our flight or fight responses. These hormones can easily trigger anxiety, irritation, and even hostility.

HSC are already prone to feelings of anxiety and depression, even without the added assistance of caffeine. Be on the lookout as you piece together how these stimulants can affect a highly sensitive child or person. The chemicals or additives in coffee, soda, sports drinks, or processed juices may elevate feelings of anxiety and over-stimulate the brain to the point of causing stress and anxiety.

Although working with their sensitivities can be particularly challenging, HSC depend on you providing them with healthy meals spaced regularly throughout the day. Being in-tuned with their emotions, you'll learn to recognize that being hungry or nutritionally unbalanced can severely mess with their moods or focus.

Another difference between non-sensitive and sensitive children is sleep. Of course, a lack of sleep causes anyone to become exhausted, stressed out, and/or unproductive. With HSC, however, not getting enough sleep can actually feel unbearable. Resting allows HSC to soothe their overstimulated senses and gives them enough energy to process their torrents of information and emotions fully.

And finally, when it comes to relationships, HSC are very particular about how they form and maintain their connections with others. They crave deep, meaningful relationships and work hard to create in-depth conversations and intimacy with their loved ones. A shallow give-and-take connection just won't do for HSP. They want to dive deep into the souls of those around them and connect in profound ways that many others might not feel comfortable with.

Many of these preferences can be similar to our own; however, with HSC, the response and processing are intricately profound. Many of us struggle to focus when we're hungry or hyped up on caffeine, but for HSP, it's even worse. We might feel cranky and tired after a poor night's sleep, but it can be grueling or seemingly insurmountable for sensitive people. Understand that their complicated and more detailed processing calls for attentive care to their preferences and needs.

THEY'RE STILL HUMAN

Despite their superpowers and wonderful gifts, highly sensitive people are still human. They have good days and bad, healthy emotions and unhealthy ones. As parents and caregivers, we must pay attention to the behaviors our highly sensitive children struggle with in order to help them thrive.

Tears are common for highly sensitive children. Their emotions are so vivid and magnified that sometimes it can be a struggle to contain them. Whether it's a heartwarming video online or a heartbreaking movie, HSC will feel (and likely display) it all.

Because of this heightened sensitivity, they're often genuinely friendly and polite. However, they might struggle with overreacting and becoming a "people pleaser" and are at risk of forgoing their own needs or emotions to make others happy. In this case, it's difficult for them to say no or set reasonable boundaries, even if it's in their best interest, as they actively try to avoid criticism.

Many people might interpret shy, introverted and people-pleasing tendencies to mean they're sweet and amazingly helpful people. Of course, this can be true. However, it doesn't mean that these people never experience negative feelings or have learned to control unhealthy emotions.

HSC are easily affected by moods and energies around them. If someone they know and spend time with is having a bad morning, this can affect how they start their day. If your stress levels are through the roof, your sensitive children are likely to mirror them in their own ways.

Because of this, along with the feeling of "otherness" they might experience, HSC are prone to depression and anxiety. These types of disorders disrupt and negatively affect their mental health.

Despite all the superhuman powers HSC might exhibit and the maturity of their emotional processing, they are still children who need love, understanding, and nurturing. They will have their good days and bad days; they'll be stronger in some areas while needing assistance in others. We, as parents and caregivers, need to remember that we are all human, experiencing life's ups and downs, and that HSC are no different in the grand scheme of humanity.

CHAPTER 3

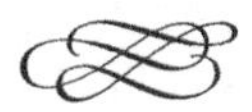

LET'S UNDERSTAND YOU

When it comes to raising children, whether you're the parent or the caregiver, you play an important role in their development. Children learn behaviors from watching you. Raising highly sensitive children means that not only is it necessary to be aware of how they function and behave, but you also need to become aware of your own emotions, actions, and behaviors, as well.

After reading the first two chapters of this book, I hope you are beginning to realize that you may also have traits of a highly sensitive person. This is great! You've probably started to understand how your own emotions and temperament have affected your highly sensitive child. To understand your highly sensitive child, you must better understand yourself.

THE HIGHLY SENSITIVE PARENT RAISING THE HIGHLY SENSITIVE CHILD

Parents or caregivers who are highly sensitive themselves may find it easier to understand highly sensitive children as their experiences may be similar. If you are highly sensitive, you will already have a basic understanding of how highly sensitive children see and process the world around them.

Highly sensitive people are generally more conscientious than non-highly sensitive individuals. They may be more aware of the consequences of choices or actions and take the time to learn how to do something the right way the first time. HSP notice warning signs quickly and are often more willing to seek out help or listen when needed.

On top of being aware of their children's emotions, highly sensitive parents are often creative and imaginative—much like their children. HSP have the ability to fully understand the uniqueness in their children and envision their child's possibilities. They're also able to understand the consequences of imposing their own creative agenda, respectfully giving them space and making it easier for them to allow their child to find their own way in their own time.

Even when parenting adolescents, an age where most parent-child communication tends to disintegrate, highly sensitive parents notice the subtle changes in their child's behavior. Highly sensitive parents can manage these mixed messages and be more flexible when it comes to their adolescent child's needs. With care and mindfulness—and a few helpful strategies—a highly sensitive parent can practice remaining calm, stable, and capable of diffusing blowups.

Highly sensitive parents will also be able to "let go" more easily than non-highly sensitive parents. Though it will still be difficult to see their child eventually leave the nest, they'll be likely to recognize when it's time for their children to find their own way.

And finally, because highly sensitive parents share the unique ability to feel things deeply, they are able to feel emotions such as pride, playfulness, and curiosity. All of this being said, there can be unique challenges for highly sensitive parents raising highly sensitive children.

For starters, children are already over-stimulating and require around-the-clock care. This can wear out highly sensitive parents, making them feel out of control or stressed out. This can be especially true when they're raising a highly sensitive child who displays large doses of intense and inflexible temperaments or is more sensation-seeking than they are.

What is the secret to being a successful highly sensitive parent? Do less to accomplish more. As a highly sensitive person, you will need time to recharge and reset in order to parent effectively and regulate your own emotions. Like all parents, you might need some extra help when it comes to raising your HSC. And that is okay!

This point cannot be emphasized enough—even if you're a non-highly sensitive parent. It is never a bad thing for any parent to ask for or receive the benefit of assistance from other people. And, if you do seek help, you don't need to explain why. As a highly sensitive parent, demonstrating that you receive support from others may even have the added benefit of modeling a positive action for your HSC that they can use in their lives.

Even if you and your highly sensitive child understand what overstimulation feels like and get equally overwhelmed, it doesn't mean that you have to face these challenges all on your own. Just as HSC need a safe haven to recharge, so do you. This will help prevent your own outbursts and assist you in regulating your own emotions. Plus, it will model for your children an effective way of dealing with high sensitivity.

Another challenge you may face is your own strong emotional reactions—both to your own life and your child's. You may feel that leaving your children to experience and deal with their emotions on their own is challenging.

Even though a child's suffering is painful for all parents, highly sensitive caregivers will feel it tenfold. Their child's sufferings could eventually become their own, making it more difficult for them to allow their child to go through the learning process they need to experience. However, a highly sensitive parent can think of this more positively; if your child is going through a difficult time, you are there to help them and learn from it so they can be more adaptable and stronger in the future.

Highly sensitive parents tend to be more emotional than caregivers who are not, and they need to be more aware of their negative emotions, especially when they are themselves overstimulated or exhausted. As a general rule, the more in control of your own emotions you are, the better. Children learn by watching us, and if you're a highly sensitive parent, this could be one of the best ways for your child to learn how to regulate their emotions and feelings. Being able to understand what it's like as a highly sensitive person gives highly sensitive parents an edge; you'll be able to effectively discuss certain episodes after they've occurred with your child and explain why they happen, as well as offer suggestions.

There are specific negative emotions that highly sensitive people are prone to that can affect and overwhelm their children. A tendency to be overly critical is one of the most important. Highly sensitive parents, though relaxed about flaws in others not close to them, tend to view their children as an extension of themselves. And, since they are more likely to be critical of their own actions, this can seep into the relationship between themselves and their children.

Even if parents don't voice their criticism, children have the uncanny ability to sense it anyway, especially if it comes in the form of disapproval. Highly sensitive parents need to accept their own unique differences and challenges in order to understand and not be critical of their children.

Guilt, another aspect of perfectionism and self-criticism, is another emotion in which highly sensitive parents can get caught up in. HSC have the capacity to think of better ways to handle things after they have occurred. That's not always a bad thing. Reviewing can assist them in improving their reactions next time. However, guilt over the past is damaging and can distract parents from moving forward positively. Critically reviewing the past can keep parents from focusing on what needs to be done in the present as well as the future.

Finally, highly sensitive parents have their own struggles with becoming overstimulated. While all parents and children can become overwhelmed, highly sensitive people feel the array of emotions sooner and stronger than most. The manner in which parents respond when their child is overwhelmed serves as a primary role model of how to deal with emotions effectively.

As a parent, when it comes to regulating emotions, you need to set a positive example. Whenever possible, show your highly sensitive child what it looks like to have your needs take precedence—to prioritize your mental health and well-being. Your child will soon realize that they will need to do the same in order to be a thriving and happy highly sensitive adult.

The best advice anyone can give to a highly sensitive parent when raising a highly sensitive child is this; pay attention to your own emotional regulation and learn to relax! Parenting requires significant amounts of understanding and sensitivity, which you already excel at as a highly sensitive parent. A loving, understanding and aware parent will raise an equally loving, understanding and aware child. It might seem difficult now, but it is worth it for you and your child.

THE NON-HIGHLY SENSITIVE PARENT RAISING THE HIGHLY SENSITIVE CHILD

If you are a non-highly sensitive adult raising a highly sensitive child, recognizing and understanding your kid can be difficult as they have different needs than your own. If you have not experienced the emotions of a highly sensitive person, you may struggle to understand the way your child thinks and reacts, but it's never too late to learn. It takes an open mind and positive attitude to maintain your relationship with a child who experiences the world more intensely and differently than you do.

As a non-highly sensitive parent, having gotten this far in the book, you have hopefully gained a basic understanding of how a highly sensitive child functions. You now know why they behave the way they do, what triggers them, and what they need in order to live as stress-free as possible. But what should you do to help your child manage their extraordinary sensitivity?

It can be difficult to understand why your child is suddenly crying over spilled milk or why they suddenly lash out after a trip to the mall. Strong emotional responses to things that do not trigger you can be difficult to handle. Strong reactions can definitely stress out a non-highly sensitive parent, as it would anyone else, but if you get revved up, your child will too. Your job is to stay calm and model emotional regulation.

When children lash out, it's usually an indication that they're feeling overstimulated or overwhelmed, and this is especially true with a highly sensitive child. Highly sensitive children also become stressed over confrontation or conflict. When you remain calm, they'll be more likely to settle down, as well.

When it comes to raising HSC, one of the most important things we need to do is acknowledge their feelings. It is important to keep acknowledgments non-judgmental, simple, and short. When children feel too much, processing all these extra words can make their feelings even more overwhelming. Even if you think your words will bring comfort, you need to recognize that adding more could have the opposite effect of what you were hoping for. A simple phrase like, "Your emotions are very large right now. Did I get that right?" is more powerful than expressing, "I see you are crying and feeling overwhelmed, and if you could just sit down and meditate, it will really help." Acknowledging their feelings allows them to get their emotions out before discussing the situation or giving solutions.

Validation is an integral part of most relationships, but especially with HSC. Like you and anyone else on earth, we all need to know that our feelings and emotions are valid, even if they might feel differently from others. As a non-highly sensitive parent, you will want to pay especially close attention to this. You might not always be able to understand why they feel the way they do—but it's essential to recognize their emotions are still valid. After your child has indicated that you understand their feelings (meaning that you asked, "Did I get that right?" or "Is there more that you want me to know?"), it is time to further validate their feelings. For example, you can add, "I see how the way your friends didn't include you made you angry. Did I get that right?"

After your child has calmed down, you can help them reflect on their behavior and emotions. Your instinct is probably to use logic to teach a lesson during the chaos, but no one wants advice when emotionally charged. In fact, the brain cannot even begin to process how to move forward until the feelings have been acknowledged as legitimate. The best lessons come from modeling and sharing your experiences empathetically. Try saying, "I understand the anger you might feel when friends leave you out. My friends have done that to me, too." Allowing the connection form between you is important. Sharing a lesson at this time can backfire and cause a disconnect with your HSC, making this worse. Your HSC needs to trust in your ability to feel with them when their emotions are ruling them.

When it comes to HSC, remember that less is more, and they will need space to regulate. It's okay to back off while still ensuring your HSC knows you're there for them. After a stressful situation, they may need time to reset and recharge before being able to socialize again—even if it's just with you. Do not take it personally—their need to be alone is about them, not a rejection of you.

It can help parents to focus on being sensitive to their sensitivity. HSC already recognize their differences, and they won't want to feel alienated from you simply due to emotional barriers. I suggest working on your own emotional sensitivity in order to understand your HSC better. Start by opening your mind to how your child is feeling. Notice and listen to their different experiences and be genuinely curious in their responses.

Highly sensitive children can be extremely hard on themselves when it comes to self-criticism. This means that you should avoid adding to that. Try to prioritize open communication when it comes to your child making mistakes or facing a difficult challenge. Engage them in conversations about possible solutions or what can be done better next time by asking their ideas. Avoid negative speech and always try to help them see the silver lining.

And finally, you will need patience. It is difficult to fully understand something we do not experience ourselves. Your job is not to always understand your highly sensitive child—this is impossible and can make your expectations of yourself too high, leading to significant frustration with yourself. Your child needs to feel accepted for who they are. Your job is to help your child adapt and develop while maneuvering between the challenges of being a highly sensitive individual.

If you find yourself struggling with patience, take a step back. Breathe in and out. Breathing out longer than breathing in triggers a physical relaxation response, is great modeling and is something you can do together. It's okay if you need a little space for yourself to reset your mind and focus. Sending yourself to a "time out" is good modeling, too, as long as you come back and don't just pretend nothing happened. Your highly sensitive child will understand. Plus, this can show them how to regulate their own stressful emotions.

Raising a highly sensitive child when you do not experience the same inflation of emotions can be difficult, but it's not impossible. Learning how your child functions and why they behave the way they do will give you an understanding of what to work on when it comes to your own behaviors.

WE CAN'T ALL BE THE SAME

Individuality and uniqueness make this world a brighter, more colorful place. We all have our own temperaments, behaviors, and habits, as well as different experiences and pasts, which make us who we are right now. Whether you're a highly sensitive individual or not, we can be stronger when we can be open to our differences.

Parents start out with a plethora of dreams and ideas about parenting. Books are bought, articles are read, and classes might even be taken. However, there may be some things that get in the way of us becoming the parents we truly want to be.

Your experiences have made you the way you are, though they do not have to define the parent you will be in the future. You might wish to be the parent who can calmly de-escalate problems without yelling but find yourself in a shouting match when your child pushes one too many buttons. Maybe you understand the reason behind this behavior—maybe not. These types of experiences can leave you feeling a bit lost about understanding yourself as a parent.

First things first: we are who we are, and we should never compare ourselves to other parents. What might work for you might not work for someone else, and vice versa. Keeping that in mind, if you ever feel as if you're letting yourself or your child down, it's time for positive self-reflection and action to replace negative reactions.

Evaluating yourself, your actions, habits, and behaviors can be a useful tool, especially when it comes to parenting a highly sensitive child. You can become more aware of how and why you think, feel, and act the way you do. Self-reflection will allow you to become more accepting, flexible and adaptive.

During self-reflection, you can identify your personal biases or preference and truly recognize them as your own work in progress. Try to identify if you are putting expectations on your own child based on your past social or cultural experiences rather than what you think they really need, or if your responses are expectations you are placing on yourself. Needless to say, we must recognize that these personal biases are not something that can define us, or we risk placing ourselves in neat, little boxes we won't be able to break out of later on. Utilizing professional support, such as a counselor or personal coach, are additional ways to help you identify and appropriately address your expectations.

Becoming more aware of ourselves as parents and caregivers allows us to become more accepting of the differences in our children, as well. It's time for us to support differences through our actions rather than just in theory. Your child may not be interested in the same things as other children, or they may be less social than you had expected them to be. But that doesn't make them any less valuable—it makes them uniquely special, a true individual with beautiful gifts to be developed and shared with the world, just like you and me.

YOUR MENTAL HEALTH

According to the National Institute of Mental Health, nearly one in five adults live with a mental illness (NIMH n.d.), so it's safe to say that many children are being raised by parents who struggle with their own mental health. Mental illnesses encompass various disorders (including depression and anxiety) that can impact an individual, their effects ranging from minimal to mild, moderate, or severe impairment.

It's important to emphasize that many parents are fully capable of raising their children while dealing with their own mental health and can give their children the stability, love and care they need. But keep in mind that identifying your own challenges is key in recognizing the consequences they are creating for your child, as well.

As a parent or caregiver, your mental health and how you deal with it are key components in raising your child. It's imperative for you to better understand your own personal challenges in order to raise your child to the best of your capabilities.

Growing up with a parent who struggles with their mental health can lead to feelings of uncertainty, anxiousness, and neglect for a child. They are likely to be right there with you experiencing the ups and downs of your mental health roller coaster, and it may feel unstable or unpredictable to them. This can be especially true for highly sensitive children.

Your highly sensitive child will be acutely attuned to your emotions—the positive and the negative—and they might struggle with coping with the wild ride your mental illness incites. If you do not exhibit healthy coping mechanisms when dealing with your mental illness, your child will also struggle to understand and learn these skills.

Children in general struggle to understand what is normal behavior and how to process these behaviors. Part of what makes this even more difficult is that, if their parents are struggling with mental health issues, most children are unaware of it. They'll take these experiences and believe them to be normal.

When we self-reflect as parents, we can come to terms with and accept our own mental health and coping mechanisms. Many adults—and parents—benefit from working with a trusted professional to assist them with new skill sets as they learn how to process their past behaviors and experiences. Ultimately, this will help you as a parent to not only improve yourself and your self-awareness but to identify and address similar concerns if your highly sensitive child exhibits symptoms of a mental illness such as depression or anxiety.

CHAPTER 4

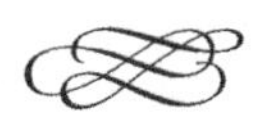

HOW TO BUILD CONFIDENCE IN YOUR HIGHLY SENSITIVE CHILD

Imagine this: you're running late for the fourth day in a row, and your child is struggling to get ready to walk out the door in time. Frustrated, you shout at your child to hurry up. The crying ensues, making everyone even later.

Your frustrated reaction is understandable. No one can really afford to be late, and children need to learn time-management strategies to succeed in both work and school. However, reacting with frustration or stress puts more focus on your own feelings rather than on how your child is feeling. Plus, adding in more stress just makes everything feel more overwhelming.

Bringing empathy and understanding can shift the dynamic noticeably. Not only will empathy allow you to acknowledge your own feelings, but it will also help you understand your child's feelings. It allows you to pause and notice what is important.

Empathy and compassion are powerful tools that give you the opportunity to understand the reason behind the behavior. These allow you to work as a team with your child to handle challenges and help create a stronger connection.

This is just one way of connecting with your child. It tells them that you understand that they are experiencing something, even when you don't exactly know how it feels. It helps validate their emotions, and, for a highly sensitive child, that's incredibly important.

When children feel validated and supported, they're likely to feel more motivated and consequently become more self-aware. Feeling supported and heard gives HSC the confidence they need to speak up about what they need and how they're feeling.

Oftentimes, people will use empathy and sympathy interchangeably; however, these are two very different concepts. When you show sympathy, you feel bad, or sorry, for the other person. Sympathy can also lead you to lower your expectations of them. It creates a sense of pity for the person and focuses on shallow feelings and statements. Sympathy can often involve a lot of judgment, whereas empathy has none. When you sympathize with someone, you understand their experience from your own perspective. Empathy, on the other hand, requires you to put yourself in their shoes, understanding why they feel this way even when you haven't experienced it yourself. With empathy, there's no need to lower expectations or be judgemental. Being empathic allows the other person to feel heard and understood. Empathy acknowledges and validates your and others' emotions.

EMPATHIZING WITH THEIR HIGHS AND LOWS

Supporting our highly sensitive children requires us to think about what it's like to be highly sensitive. One such way we can empathize with our HSC is by understanding that they might become overwhelmed and will need a safe space to retreat to after an over-stimulating event. Having the foresight to schedule a break in a quiet space is a great way of showing your child that you understand and empathize with their needs.

When it comes to HSC, parents and caregivers must prepare for everything—especially dramatic and recurrent highs and lows. As with many parenting concepts, the same can be said for non-highly sensitive children, but as you know, HSC have extreme ups and downs. When you empathize with the inevitability of highs and lows, you help prepare yourselves for the new experiences and challenges you will face in life.

For example, if your highly sensitive child is about to start a new school, bringing them for a visit before classes start helps them get used to the new environment and meet their new teacher. This prepares them to handle the change they might not welcome or want. Some highly sensitive children might struggle with how to react in different social situations. You can help them by role-playing different scenarios to give them some practice. When it comes to dealing with their intense emotions, try providing your child with a toolkit of ideas—breathing exercises, using fidget tools to calm their nerves, or other ways to mentally reset. This will help them develop the necessary skill sets they will need to self-manage their own emotions even when you are not around.

For older children, this could simply be penciling in some downtime between events in their busy schedules. Take the time to teach them about healthy boundaries that will help them process their emotions safely. For example, non-highly sensitive children might have no problem going from a sports practice straight to another social event. But a highly sensitive child might need some time to reset in between as both scenarios require a lot of emotional and physical energy.

Another thing to note is that HSC are extremely conscious of hypocrisy. Approach discipline carefully, even more so than you probably would with non-sensitive children. Simply saying "Because I said so!" won't necessarily work with your highly sensitive child. For example, you might tell your child that they are not allowed to use certain bad words, but they hear you say them. It might be tempting to respond with a quick and easy "Because I'm an adult..." but in this situation, it will seem hypocritical to a highly sensitive child.

As parents and caregivers, our first response is often to offer help and try to rescue our children when they feel distressed. However, offering help implies the judgment that they cannot do it themselves. When you think about "help" in this context, you can begin to understand and address their needs differently. Judgment is a huge disservice to your highly sensitive child. It prevents them from learning how to handle difficult situations on their own rather than figuring it out for themselves. Instead, we should use our empathy to understand their ups and downs and teach them how to effectively manage their emotions, giving them the skills to handle whatever life throws at them now and in the future.

RISE ABOVE

One of the most important things we need to survive in this world is flexibility. Flexibility helps us get through difficult events we cannot predict or control. Flexibility allows us to work effectively in teams and develop healthy relationships. Unfortunately, HSC often struggle with being adaptive and flexible. Learning to be flexible can be harder for HSC due to their low sensory thresholds.

HSC already live in a world of overwhelming stimuli that can make them feel more out of control than non-highly sensitive children. To cope with their constant state of high alert, HSC depend on fixed expectations to make their daily lives feel bearable and manageable. It's often difficult for them to accept spontaneously presented alternative ways of doing things.

The more they feel a lack of control over their environment, the more controlling they can become in other ways. This can result in the need for HSC to have a specific plate for dinner, only tolerate one color of cup, be ridgid about what clothes they will or will not wear, or arrange their food so that items don't mix on their plate. These are all examples of control opportunities that translate into coping mechanisms HSC can utilize to create a feeling of consistency and calm in their lives.

We can help our HSC to become flexible and adaptive by being understanding of the reasons why they need to create control. For starters, we can repeat what we hear and then validate their feelings and experiences. It's important to remember that the *feelings* themselves are not the problem; it's their *reactions* that can become problematic. However, when you acknowledge the driving feelings behind the behaviors, you and your child will be better equipped to handle them in more effective and healthy ways.

When setting limits and boundaries for your highly sensitive child, it's always best to do so calmly and lovingly. Helping them understand the "why" behind the sudden change or unexpected direction helps them feel a sense of control. Show your child that you are willing to engage in positive ways rather than continue a negative back-and-forth dynamic. For example, if the child's mother comes to pick up their highly sensitive child rather than dad, they might feel upset and react negatively because that's not what they expected. Instead of arguing with them, it's best to calmly explain and then move on to positive distractions such as playing their favorite song in the car or telling a funny story.

When you set boundaries and refuse to engage in negative demands or behaviors, you're showing your child what it's like to see the world from other people's perspectives. This helps your child understand other people's needs and emotions even when they are overwhelmed by their own.

Sharing is a core behavior when it comes to child development. However, your highly sensitive child can struggle to recognize that other children want a turn. Calmly explaining that it is kind and empathetic to give other children a turn and praising them for waiting is just one way to reinforce good and positive behavior in a healthier way.

And finally, modeling the behavior you want to teach is always an excellent course of action. As you go about your day, highlight the times you need to be flexible with your child. If something unexpected happens during your daily routine, model how to handle this change and discuss it with your child. Not only will they be able to see how they should behave when it comes to unpredictable changes, but they will be able to understand why they must be flexible.

When your highly sensitive child follows what you've modeled, acknowledge it and give positive feedback. Catching your child in the act of doing it correctly is an incredibly powerful teaching technique with HSC. Catching them in the act of doing something right reinforces the flexibility you're trying to teach them. You can also point out the benefits of being flexible, especially if your child is old enough to understand. Show and tell them why it would be good for them to participate in the changes they might face.

THE NORMALIZATION MISTAKE

As you may have experienced, a highly sensitive child likely has difficulties navigating the social jungle. Many people do not understand the unique traits of a highly sensitive child. As they get involved with social events, school, and group activities, your own child will recognize that they are different from their peers and friends. Although this is a challenge, this isn't necessarily a bad thing.

One of the biggest mistakes is trying to force your unique child into conforming to what is considered by others to be "normal." In this world, there really isn't any such thing—we're all different in our own ways. Yet, with the often competitive standards for scoring performance in schools, measuring kids against each other in communities, looming societal performance expectations and, of course, the ever-present pressure of social media, we're told that there is somehow a "norm" that should be followed and adhered to.

But here's the thing: trying to force your child to conform to social norms will probably just cause more problems than before, and it will certainly diminish the very things that make them special. There is nothing wrong with being sensitive or reacting with emotion.

When it comes to discipline, parents of HSC might find additional challenges to deal with beyond those of non-highly sensitive children. Here are a few things to understand to avoid trying to "normalize" our unique children.

Don't just accept their sensitivity. Embrace and applaud it. This is an integral part of who they are. Rather than discouraging your child from feeling these big emotions, it's best to emphasize their strengths.

Acknowledge that what might come easy for other children might not be so for them. When you're feeling frustrated, remember that this sensitivity makes them extremely compassionate and empathetic to others.

Also, set limits when it comes to discipline. As much as you'd like to give in to avoid upsetting your highly sensitive child, it won't be beneficial for them. For example, if your child throws a tantrum when you tell them to turn off video games, it could be tempting to give them "just five more minutes" to settle them. However, this encourages inappropriate behavior and lets them know that if they push your buttons just enough, they will get what they want despite the rules and limits you've set. It's important to be flexible while still maintaining the level of discipline they need to become responsible adults. The constant giving in will not help prepare them for the "real world" later on. Consistent, reasonable rules will give them plenty of room to be themselves within respectful and healthy boundaries.

Like most people, HSC respond better to encouragement and praise than negativity. Positive parenting should continue even when your child is unsuccessful, though be sure that whatever encouragement you give is genuine and earned. Praising your highly sensitive child for something "normal" children are expected to do will not have the effect you're looking for. We don't want to highlight the "otherness" they might already be feeling. If they accomplish something other children do, then that's great! But we shouldn't point it out more than we would to any other child. The difference between praise and powerful encouragement can be difficult for parents to understand.

For example, if your child struggled with learning to tie their shoes on their own longer than others, try to avoid making a big deal about how they finally did it. Instead, praise them for a job well done just as you would for the child who learned this skill in an average time frame.

Don't give up; talk to other parents and professionals and acknowledge that finding the right methods to discipline a highly sensitive child can be challenging and varied at times. Some parents might even avoid it altogether to sidestep the waterfall of emotions and reduce their child's pain. However, it's critical to discipline HSC; they need boundaries just like all children to help them grow and develop into capable adults.

QUENCHING INFERIORITY

Life can be especially hard for HSC, and, as noted before, they'll often try to take control over certain areas in their lives just to feel stable.

According to the American Psychological Association's Dictionary of Psychology (APA), an inferiority complex is a "basic feeling of inadequacy and insecurity, deriving from actual or imagined physical or psychological deficiency." At some point in our lives, we worry about our abilities and, though it can be distressing, it's normal for us to question how we compare to those around us. For most, these feelings of insufficiency are situational or occasional. For HSC, they can be extreme.

They might already be aware of their differences and compare themselves to their friends and peers. On top of all that, they can be prone to developing an inferiority complex. They may respond differently to events that create chronic low self-esteem. They might focus on their shortcomings, become critical of themselves and attack their own self-esteem. They may become frequently irritated, try to act over-smart or perhaps they might even stammer when talking or avoid making eye contact during conversations.

We can help combat these unhealthy responses in several different ways. The first way, as always, is to accept them as they are. Having unreasonable expectations for your child puts them at risk of developing an inferiority complex. Rather than pushing them to develop more external traits, accept and help them discover their more intrinsic qualities. Remember, expectations lead to resentments for both you and your child.

Avoid comparing your highly sensitive child to others. Comparisons do nothing but make them feel less worthy or that they will need to change to fit in. It can be demotivating, even if you're comparing them to their siblings as a form of motivation. Especially for HSC, but really for most children, it is not as motivating as you might think.

If you've noticed some of the signs that your child might be struggling with an inferiority complex, spending time with them is crucial. Talk to your child and genuinely listen to what they want to share with you. Opening up the lines of communication will encourage a stronger bond where they will feel more comfortable discussing problems with you.

Be mindful to avoid scolding your child in front of other people. It's fairly common for children to have small fights with each other, and it's part of human nature to complain from time to time. Before you take any action, take a moment to listen to your child. If they are in the wrong, it would be better to pull them aside and chat with them privately rather than in front of their friends. Children are quick to blame and point fingers, and punishing them in public will only make your child an easier target or stronger aggressor. These public humiliations might have a detrimental effect on their mental health and mental state overall, as well. It won't help them improve their relationships with you or their friends. Remember, all they can hear when you are upset is that they are bad and wrong—emphasizing the negative only enhances it and never creates a positive learning experience.

When you need to have a chat with your highly sensitive child, it will help if you share some of your own experiences—both your successes and your failures. This will teach them that they are not alone and that everyone struggles with something or that others might excel in certain areas more than their friends, family or peers. And you will *always* want to give positive feedback and encouragement to boost their confidence.

When giving feedback, stay positive and avoid criticizing your children. You should only give criticism in the most extreme cases. Always keep your words and attitude positive when talking to your child about their mistakes or mess-ups. Parenting is tough, and sometimes, we might not even realize what sort of effect our words can have on our children. Keep in mind that your goal is to understand and positively support your child.

It is essential to understand the difference between praise and encouragement. Praise is non-specific. For example, praise is saying "great job!" without clarifying what you liked about the job. Powerful encouragement is more specific, such as noting the beautiful tone on the last note of their music practice. Praise can sometimes feel vague and lacking, whereas encouragement allows your child to fully understand just what they've done so they can repeat similar actions or behavior in the future.

If you've noticed that your child's confidence and self-esteem are dipping, despite your best efforts to motivate and encourage them, it's always a good choice to seek out professional help. Early intervention can make all the difference in the world as you and your child navigate these developmental challenges. Remember, expanding your child's resources in life is a positive reflection on your parenting skills. If they need it, give it.

THE COMPASSIONATE WAY TO HANDLE OVERSTIMULATION

Children grow by interacting with a stimulating environment they can explore; it's an important part of their development. But, here again, these environments might be too much for HSC, and they may become overstimulated and distressed.

Overstimulation occurs when children experience a tidal wave of sensations, sounds, or activities that they cannot easily cope with. For example, your highly sensitive child might become easily overstimulated in a crowd where there is a lot of noise and action. This can make them feel tired and cranky. As you understand this, these outbursts can be accepted as your child's way of communicating to you that they need a break.

Some signs that your child might be overstimulated include becoming more hyper, aggressive or overexcited. Or they might go in the complete opposite direction and zone out, withdraw or retreat. Your understanding is key as your HSC learns how to deal with these crushing feelings and develops the communication skills they need to tell you how they feel.

The key to helping your child in these situations is to pay attention to their behaviors in different scenarios. For your highly sensitive child, some stimuli might become more overbearing than others. Recognizing the early signs and the situations that bring them about will be helpful for you in intervening positively before your child breaks down.

Utilizing any activity that requires them to move their bodies is usually positively pro-active. Playing simple games such as "Simon Says" helps calm their bodies and reset their minds as they focus on the exercise. This type of activity provides distraction as well as an opportunity for feelings of focused control, providing balance with overwhelming stimuli.

When possible, try preventing overstimulation by developing a balance between activities and downtime. A child's brain develops faster in the first few years of their life than at any other time. This is when their brain will be working hard to process all the different sounds, sights, smells, and tastes around them, creating millions and millions of connections.

Try to avoid cramming their schedule with activity after activity and plan a few slots per day in which they can simply relax. I'm sure they're not the only ones who might need a break. Unstructured free time is an important habit to incorporate into the constant rush of our daily lives, and it's crucial for highly sensitive children to have downtime throughout their day.

On the other hand, if you have begun to rearrange your entire daily schedule to deal with your child's overstimulation, it might be a sign to seek professional help. If your child's overstimulated outbursts become too frequent or extreme, start with your healthcare provider or trusted expert and seek additional insights into how to effectively integrate whatever further resources your child might need.

Keep in mind that there isn't a perfect amount of stimulation or a set amount for when it becomes too much. Each child is different, and you know your child better than anyone else. Learn to understand your child's signs and try to give them as much downtime as they might need throughout the day.

EMPATHY, SUPPORT, AND RESPECT

In addition to increased understanding, I hope you have found encouragement in some of the suggestions shared in the previous chapters. I've discussed ways to support, empathize with, and care for your highly sensitive child. Of course, you can find many other approaches to give both you and your child the support you need. Once you've started to understand your child's temperament, it will become natural for you to open up discussions with your highly sensitive child about their strengths and how unique they are. This will magnify their confidence in you, lift their own self confidence and inspire them to continue being the best they can be.

Yet, it isn't just support for them that is necessary. *You* also need support. If you're a highly sensitive person raising a highly sensitive kid, you might be just as attuned to their emotions as they are to yours. This can cause burnout or unnecessary stress and can potentially inhibit your child's own learning in how to handle their emotions or challenges. Seeking out support for yourself will always benefit both you and your child.

If you're not a highly sensitive person, it's still a good idea to seek outside resources when helpful or necessary. You will inevitably have times when you feel frustrated with the challenges that come with raising HSC, and you might not fully understand your child's struggles or obstacles. Finding support from a trusted professional, family member or friend can help you process your own feelings and identify positive solutions for your next steps.

And, just as you might need support from others, your child will need something similar as well. Playdates and informal group activities provide interactions that help create a supportive friend network with deep, meaningful connections. Your modeling these kinds of activities and relationships with your child will give them the ability to benefit from supportive, loving and caring relationships with their peers.

Lastly, be collaborative. You are not alone and, as the famous saying goes, sometimes it takes a village. Your child will have lots of adults in their lives; teachers, coaches, babysitters and other family members. If you help them understand your child's temperament, they will also be able to help your child grow and develop as a highly sensitive person.

CHAPTER 5

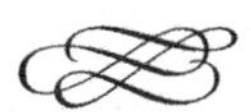

THE FULL GUIDE TO COMPASSION AND EMPATHY

Highly sensitive children need guidance and support from early on. You can help them strike a balance between how they view the world and how they react by keeping your reactions neutral. Expressions of neutrality are neither good nor bad but can help your highly sensitive child grow into a well-functioning adult who knows how to regulate and understand their feelings.

Yet again, remember that as you expand your knowledge, understanding, and resource base, your child will not only develop and grow but thrive as well. When you have a better understanding of your feelings, your child will too. Your child will often mirror you as they grow, following what you do, saying what you say. Of course, you want this mirror to be the most healthy, loving, and intelligent reflection possible.

HSC are not bad kids or wrong in any way when it comes to their emotions. Think of the times you've been overwhelmed to your breaking point—remember how difficult it was for you to regulate those feelings. This situation has probably even happened to you recently. As an adult, it feels difficult. Imagine what it must feel like for a child to experience this almost every day. Fine-tuning your understanding and compassion will soothe the frustration and grow the peaceful connection you hope to have.

SUPPORTING YOUR HIGHLY SENSITIVE CHILD

You can help support your child in various ways and guide them to navigate their emotions. For starters, you can help them understand "feeling" words and how to describe their emotions. Children struggle with handling their emotions when they cannot accurately communicate their frustration. By sharing some of your own feelings, both the good and the bad, you can help your child identify and communicate their emotions effectively.

Talk to your child about their feelings and experiences frequently. Don't shy away from what might feel like an uncomfortable discussion around emotions and reactions. Be confident and concise in these discussions, knowing they will be helpful to you and your child. Remember, timing is everything. Wait until you and your child are calm before discussing what happened. Take it slow—one question at a time with acknowledgement, clarification and a pause. Inquire as to how the event made them feel. Then, brainstorm with them about how they can deal with similar events and emotions in the future.

Teaching your child breathing techniques that they can use can be a good idea for when things get stressful or out of hand. Although this might seem obvious, you might forget to take the time to slow down and simply take a breath of fresh air for yourself. Teach your child how to pause and take calming breaths to help settle their nerves and mind. Take time together to focus on breathing techniques, allowing you both to slow down and practice as well as share the experience. Remind your child that breathing helps us train our body's reactions to stressful situations. It also helps decrease the production of harmful stress hormones. Slow breathing activates our parasympathetic reaction, causing us to calm down. Our bodies trigger a relaxation response when we exhale longer than we inhale. Practicing this physiological response with your child is a valuable approach to teaching them how to manage themselves when overwhelmed or overstimulated.

Make sure that you promote a relationship that allows your

highly sensitive child to feel validated and understood. To others around them, they might be labeled "too emotional" or "sensitive" and therefore ostracized from their friends or peers. Perhaps they've even had other family members make negative comments about some of their unique traits. Combat this with discussions and actions that communicate ways that will enable your HSC to feel more understood and accepted.

At some point in our lives we have been told to contain our emotions, such as crying in public. We've probably been told that many emotions are deemed "unhealthy," like frustration, anger or hurt. However, our HSC experience this entire spectrum of human emotions twice over. When we tell our children that their emotions are valid and acceptable, we're letting them know that it's okay to experience them—that these emotions aren't "bad" and that they can learn how to cope with them in a healthy manner. Then, we give them the tools they will need to transform these emotions into constructive feelings and actions.

HSC are incredibly sensitive to feelings of injustice. How other people are treated affects them greatly. Understanding that this is a compassionate, loving response rather than an overreaction is key. Assure your child that it is healthy to experience strong emotions when it comes to injustice, that the world needs people to care about others just as they do. Use this opportunity to help them take meaningful action about the topic that has upset them. Help them find a volunteer or donation activity that will turn their feelings of pain or compassion into something productive, giving them confidence, motivation and positive feelings of helping.

You will also want to make sure that your highly sensitive child understands that it is okay to let people know when they need alone time. Sometimes, it can be extremely hard saying "no" as a highly sensitive person because HSC feel the need to please those around them. They need to learn that it is perfectly acceptable to set boundaries to maintain their mental health and to take a break when needed. Many adults still struggle with this, but the earlier you teach your child, the easier it will be later on. Let them know they have the power to say "no."

In this day and age, it feels like the world is in a constant state of go-go-go. Many of us struggle to find time for ourselves, let alone time to really process our emotions. We tend to forget that, as humans, we do actually need time to process the constant stream of information we are subjected to. Again, HSC are likely to need even more time to address this need. Their depth of processing can be deeper than the oceans, and they often feel the need to analyze information from every possible angle before connecting it to a bigger picture. When this happens, be patient and give your child the time they need to process the world around them.

Most importantly of all, remind your highly sensitive child that they are important to the world as well as to you and your family. Most people agree that the world could use more empathy and understanding. Your child possesses those qualities. Keep reminding them how their sensitivity and love are gifts that could help change the whole world someday—because it is, and it will!

EARLY START PAYS OFF

When we think about emotional intelligence, we often assume that this is solely a skill saved for adulthood, or at least an age where we are able to think about feelings more in-depth. However, emotional intelligence actually begins in childhood. Having strong and well-developed emotional intelligence is key to successful relationships throughout life—both interpersonal and social.

Emotional intelligence refers to a persons' ability to identify and express their feelings in constructive ways. There are five pillars to teaching emotional intelligence: self-awareness, self-regulation, internal motivation, empathy, and social skills (Goleman 2020). These five concepts can be taught at any age in various ways that are age-appropriate. We covered how to help your child build more self-awareness in Chapter Four—teaching them to recognize their mistakes and accept themselves for who they truly are. In the next few sections and chapters, we will go more in-depth into how we can help our highly sensitive children self-regulate their emotions while instilling confidence, maintaining empathy and enhancing social skills.

Emotions and feelings are so universal, many adults sometimes assume that children are naturally aware of—and can identify—feelings. However, just as we learned to walk, run, and play, we also learned about emotions as we developed. Understanding people's emotions is just like any other vital skill in our social and emotional development—and just as it's important to teach children the basics of right and wrong when they're young, it's essential to teach them about their emotions, as well.

So, why is talking about feelings so important? Children who can understand their own emotions as well as others' can regulate their reactions to strong feelings. Although their emotional intelligence might depend on their age, it's always important for them to recognize and understand different feelings.

For example, most of us probably have started to teach our children how to share, even when they're extremely young. The concept of sharing is one lesson most young children learn in school or even at home with their siblings. It helps them become more aware of others around them and allows them to develop social skills.

As parents and caregivers, emotional intelligence is one of the best tools we can assist our HSCs in developing—and while academic skills are certainly important, emotional intelligence is vital for our children as they successfully maneuver through life's obstacles. Emotional intelligence helps each of us cultivate the best versions of ourselves.

BUILDING RESILIENCE IN A SENSITIVE CHILD

Resilience is the ability to adapt to adversity, trauma, threats, and other challenges that are sources of stress. Resilience is a skill that can be taught and learned. Resilience does not mean your child will never face difficulty or stress—it just means they will have internal tools to deal with situations outside of their control.

One way of fostering resilience is by teaching your child the importance of connecting with their friends and peers, as well as family. Connecting with others gives us the social support we need and allows us to build upon our resilience. Facing any challenge alone can be difficult, but the support of family and friends gives us the reinforcement we need to get through it.

Highly sensitive children often feel out of control when it comes to their stimulant-filled lives. Help them feel more in control by teaching them to help others. HSC will feel empowered by engaging in age-appropriate volunteer work or even just helping you around the house. Ask your child to come up with their own ideas for ways they can help their friends and teachers at school.

In addition to breathing exercises, there are many other ways for your child to become resilient. For example, teaching them about self-care, including making time to eat properly, exercise, and getting enough sleep, can ensure that their lives and bodies stay balanced and better able to deal with stress. To take care of difficult situations, they must first be taking care of themselves, which is a necessary skill that will be invaluable throughout their lives.

You can also teach your child the importance of establishing goals. Helping them set reasonable and attainable objectives toward these goals helps them move forward one step at a time. When there is a significant challenge that feels like too big of an obstacle, help your HSC identify smaller, achievable steps that move them closer to their goals without feeling overwhelmed.

Finally, all children need to learn how to accept change. Routines and habits are particularly helpful for HSC. They help them maneuver through life more easily. However, life isn't always predictable, and routines can change without warning. Help your child understand that even though change can be scary, it's a part of life and can be handled just like anything else.

The road to resilience is a personal journey. Use your own experiences and knowledge to understand and guide your children on their own paths. The key is finding what works for both you and your child. What might work for others might not work for you or your own highly sensitive kid. Don't give up. Teach them and show them how to cope with life's ups and downs.

RESPECTING THE INDIVIDUAL CHILD

Respect is vital when it comes to relationships. Without it, negative feelings such as resentment can develop. Think back to how you felt when someone did not respect you. That memory of the experience probably does not incite the most pleasant of feelings.

There are several ways we can show our own children the respect and dignity they truly deserve to help create more positive future experiences. As adults, it can be easy to forget that children deserve the same respect and dignity as anyone else. This is often evident in the way adults interrupt a child or talk over them, dismiss what a child has to say, or physically touch them without asking for consent. While these might be common behaviors in adults, they tell a child they are not seen or respected.

Recently, there has been a broader recognition of the importance of allowing children to make choices about their own bodies. Children should have the right to choose whether or not they feel comfortable enough to hug someone, even if it is a close family member. This goes hand in hand with encouraging them to set their own boundaries and learning to say "no" when they need to (without feeling guilty). Allowing them the right to choose what to do with their body will have a huge effect on how they feel about their autonomy and their ability to stand up for themselves in the future.

When interacting with your child, remember to use good manners. It may sound ridiculous but think about it. How do we greet our friends? Our neighbors? Would we allow someone to use bad manners towards us? If not, we need to model this behavior to our children. Not only will you show them the proper way to treat others, but you will also be teaching them how to respect themselves.

I've mentioned before how sharing can be a great way to develop emotional intelligence, but we should be careful in how we do it. We do not want to force our children to share. Instead, we should actively encourage them and reward them for sharing when they want to. Allow them to choose when they would like to share, and respect their "no" when they do not. This is important because it teaches our children to really think about why they would want to share, rather than blindly following rules others lay out for them or becoming people pleasers. It gives them a choice and allows them to truly understand their own actions.

When we force our children to share, they might not understand the reason behind the action and therefore not integrate sharing into their values. They know it's good and that their parents expect it, but commanding it does not allow them to make that choice for themselves. It also takes away their autonomy, their right to choose whether they wish to share with others and their ability to create empathy for others.

This next tip might be a little more difficult, but we should always respond to their fumbles with comfort and grace. To us, it might be adorable if our child accidentally puts their shirt on inside out or if they take a slight tumble in the soft grass. However, children are quick to pick up on being patronized, especially HSC, even if we don't mean it to come out that way. It could be humiliating and demoralizing, especially if they don't understand why you find it to be funny in the first place. Instead, treat their mistakes, even the funny ones, as you would any adult—give them a genuine smile and help them correct them respectfully. This can help teach them that it's all right to make mistakes and that they shouldn't be afraid to slip up now and then.

Allowing them to make mistakes with grace encourages them

to be more independent, which is the goal. If your child wants to do something on their own, such as dressing themselves or feeding themselves, then that's great! Allowing them to do independent tasks on their own will boost their confidence and increase their ability. The best way to learn, after all, is by doing.

Finally—and I know this is incredibly difficult—we need to respect their privacy. Most parents love retelling cute stories of their children, even if those stories might be embarrassing or personal. Your child might not want to hear that story being retold or fear that story getting around to people they know. Showing respect for their private life will solidify the trust between you, which is an essential part of any relationship. As they continue to grow and you continue to respect that privacy, you will develop a stronger bond because you're showing that you are honest, reliable and respectful.

WHAT CONFIDENCE MEANS FOR YOUR CHILD

Having confidence is an important aspect of your child's development. Confidence is the belief in our own abilities; it allows us to face challenges throughout our lives. Children with a strong sense of self-confidence feel excited to learn new things and have less fear of the unknown. Confidence provides an inner sense of stability and capability that we all need to thrive.

Confidence is also vital for getting along with others and maneuvering through the multitude of social challenges children face as part of growing up. Self-confidence is a learned emotional behavior built upon a child's perceptions, experiences and interactions. Self-confidence is largely shaped by parents, caregivers and teachers.

Confidence is not consistent across situations. Your child may feel more confident in certain situations than others. For example, a child with a lot of energy and athleticism might feel more confident at a sports event than in a classroom. If your child really enjoys math, they might have more self-confidence in the classroom. Having confidence requires courage, and we cannot feel confident if we are not courageous enough to get out of our comfort zones.

There are many benefits to having confidence. For example, having self-confidence boosts performance. Whether your child is great at answering math problems or loves to read, self-confidence is the key to their ability to excel in those areas.

Confidence enhances social skills and allows children to interact with others and develop deeper connections. Self-confidence helps children become more resilient, enabling them to bounce back faster and motivating them to get through tough challenges.

HOW TO INSTILL CONFIDENCE SAFELY AND PERMANENTLY

One of the best ways to instill confidence in your child is by establishing routines. When daily events are predictable, it gives your child a sense of control over their world, and they feel safe, confident, and stable by knowing what to expect. Unpredictability can cause anxiety—especially for a highly sensitive child. Random routines can make their daily lives scary, preventing them from exploring and learning effectively. When a child is distressed, they can not focus on anything other than protecting themselves and finding safety and stability. For example, a child who is constantly moved from one unstable home to another is likely to find it hard to concentrate on schoolwork and their development.

Children develop their identity and a sense of self-confidence through play and exploration. While highly sensitive children need breaks now and then to recharge, play is also an important component of their development. Allowing your child to lead during playtime helps them build their self-confidence, helps them develop leadership skills and gives them a positive sense of assertiveness.

While you want to instill independence in them, you also want to help them become strong, confident problem solvers. You can do this by supporting them through problems rather than completely solving them. When your child begins to feel frustrated, you may find yourself wanting to save them and complete the task for them. Instead, offer your own observations of the problem at hand and then ask if they can identify what is causing the problem and what ideas for solutions they have. Your confidence in their ability to come up with solutions on their own supercharges their confidence. It also gets their critical thinking skills going so they can solve the challenge on their own while learning new ways to think of solutions.

Helping a child feel useful and helpful is another great way to build their confidence. Try giving your child age-appropriate tasks or chores they can do independently or help you with. This can be anything from helping sort laundry to feeding the family pet or picking up after themselves. Feeling more responsible and accomplishing the tasks correctly will solidify their confidence in doing these actions in the future.

When it comes to difficult tasks, encourage your child to figure them out in their own way rather than doing it for them. For example, if they want to try and tie their shoes on their own but have not yet learned how, give them the chance to work it out rather than jumping straight in. You can break down the tasks into manageable, smaller steps for them to work through. Let them know you believe in their capabilities to achieve this goal and try to communicate that you will not be disappointed if they make a mistake or aren't ready for this challenge just yet. Constant support and encouragement can be the building blocks for achieving confidence.

Another way to instill confidence is to practice positive self-talk and affirmations. The development of self-affirmations is supported by neuroscientific research. MRI evidence suggests that neural pathways are increased when individuals practice affirmations regularly (Cascio et al. 2016). Highly sensitive children, as noted before, are prone to self-criticism and extreme negative feelings if they do something less than perfect. We can help them combat negative self-talk by brainstorming together how to rephrase negative thoughts into something positive.

Affirmations such as "I am an amazing kid" or "I will be confident and fearless today" can help reset negativity. I recommend picking one or two lines that are easy for them to remember. Whenever they are feeling down about themselves or not feeling very confident, have them repeat those lines. Once these affirmations become a habit, you might find that your child will start believing in those words and themselves. Keep the affirmation simple, and let your child find the words.

Building self-confidence does not happen overnight. It's a long process that requires conscious effort from both you and your child. However, if you follow the above tips, you will see your child grow more confident over time. You might even find that your confidence grows along with your child's.

CHAPTER 6

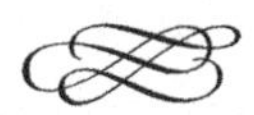

RESPONDING WITH LOVE (LOVE NEVER FAILS)

One of the most vital influences of every child's growth and development is their attachment to parents and caregivers. Highly sensitive children especially need to feel a deep connection with their primary attachment figures. Research has shown that HSC are more affected than their non-highly sensitive counterparts by attachment. To thrive, they need nurturing and supportive environments, which include the types of relationships they have with the primary caregivers in their lives.

HSC are often highly intelligent. Many can understand what you teach them, even from an early age, so it's important to coach them in emotional matters to help them achieve balance. In this chapter, we will discuss how to support and guide your highly sensitive child into becoming a capable and independent adult.

EMOTIONAL COACHING FOR THE HIGHLY SENSITIVE CHILD

Emotional sensitivity can be measured using two different scales. The first measures how in-tune your child is to their own emotions. Some children may feel things very deeply, while others may not understand what they are feeling or may even be unaware of their emotions. The second scale measures how tuned-in your child is to others' emotions. Some kids can be very aware of what is going on with others, while some may find it difficult to respond to what they see around them appropriately.

As noted, each child is different regarding their high sensitivity. Some can be high on one scale while low on the other. Your child could very well be aware of their own emotions while not fully aware of others' feelings, and vice versa. To identify your child's level of awareness of their feelings, consider the following questions using a scale of one through five in the range from "unaware of feelings" to "feels strongly:"

- Is your child able to express their emotions and feelings clearly?
- Is your child prone to crying often, and do they have a hard time letting go of things?
- Does your child get overly upset when someone criticizes, disciplines or makes negative comments towards them?

To find the level of their sensitivity to others' emotions, ask the following questions:

- Does your child notice when others are hurt or upset?
- Do they seem to mirror what others around them are feeling?
- Does your child show empathy and sympathy to others who are feeling upset?

Again, number one on the scale represents insensitivity toward others' feelings, while five represents emotionally tuned in. If most of your responses fall toward five, then this is an indicator that your child is emotionally sensitive. They will tend to display their emotions in a more straightforward way, oftentimes more dramatically.

Taking your child's sensitivity into account and understanding that it is an important part of their temperament is a critical step in creating positive interactions with your child. Depending on the types of sensitivity you are addressing, you can accomplish this in various ways. For example, if the issue is over clothing and conflict about dressing, consider taking your child shopping to find clothes that feel comfortable to them, respectfully understanding the physical and emotional feelings they have with some clothing. You can also give them time in the morning, or the night before, to make their own choices and feel sure their clothes will feel comfortable for their day.,

One step that might seem obvious, but can be easily overlooked, is to avoid labeling your child with any negativity. Calling them things such as a "whiner" or "selfish," or even telling them they need to get thicker skin can all be detrimental to their mental health rather than helping them become stronger. Instead, use positive words and phrases such as "caring and loving" or remind them that they are "aware of their feelings" and how good that is for them.

Send them messages that help them appreciate how unique and incredible they are. Explain to them that they express emotions strongly and that that's not a bad thing. Remind them how much they care for others and that they can acknowledge their emotions for themselves and others before moving on. Work as a team to understand their temperament and create strategies together on how to deal with their intense emotions.

Often when children are upset, it's because they need us to understand their emotions, hear them out, and empathize or somehow relate—i.e., legitimize what they are feeling. This alone can help them feel calmer and more settled, and often there won't be a need to solve a problem. Of course, sometimes, children will truly need help with problem-solving, and we can teach and guide them by helping them work it out step by step.

HOW TO COMMUNICATE YOUR UNDYING LOVE

Children, whether highly sensitive or not, need love, time, and attention. As a parent or caregiver, you have the most lasting influence on their lives and it's up to you to help build their confidence and nurture their self-love. When it comes to highly sensitive children, daily routines help them feel more stable and secure and will have the most impact on their behaviors. There are a few things you can consider adding to your daily routines with your highly sensitive child.

As always, we should strive to understand what our children are comfortable with. Some children find it upsetting to be touched, while others crave physical contact. Whether it is hugs and kisses or air bumps and laughter, our children depend on and thrive on the continuous reminders of our love. This might seem like a no-brainer, but in the hustle and bustle of our day, we might slip past maintaining our love-showing routine actions simply for the sake of saving time. However, studies have shown that showering warmth and affection on our children positively correlates to higher levels of confidence, self-esteem, better communication, and lower levels of behavioral problems (Child Trends n.d.).

Another great idea to add to your weekly or daily routines is to take a drive together. Even if it might mean your "to-do" list will take just a bit longer to complete than planned, the time and conversation you can have, in a car, with your child will be worth it. Asking your child to assist with chores or outings tells them that you appreciate their involvement and helps them feel needed. Car rides also provide a neutral territory and unthreatening environment for diffusing difficult situations.

Throwing unexpected, thoughtful and fun activities into your usual routine helps make your child feel important and loved. For example, you could send them a "snail mail" letter just for a surprise. Receiving physical letters is so rare these days that it's sure to make your child feel even more special.

You could also plan short trips with small groups or as a family to spend more fun, special time together. Visiting museums, parks, zoos, or the library can be extra special to your child if their interests are understood and prioritized. If you go to the library, let your child pick out a few books you could read together to spend even more quality time with them.

Giving your children the fun, love and attention they crave will help them grow and develop into more confident, secure, and capable adults.

Parenting isn't just about hard work and teaching skills. These years go by pretty fast, so take the time to treasure them and create lasting relationships and memories for your children and yourself.

DISCIPLINING IN LOVE

While discipline is an essential part of raising children, it can often be a struggle for highly sensitive children, especially with their unique ability to feel emotions more extremely than others. They are easily overwhelmed and will be prone to crying as well as worrying about getting into trouble. They require a lot of reassurance.

In addition, not only are they extra sensitive to emotions, but to physical triggers as well. Things such as raised voices, sharp changes in tone, and negative criticism can easily and acutely affect them. While some children might require strict discipline, using harsh and negative punishments are likely to cause more problems with your highly sensitive child.

In fact, positive punishment and positive reinforcement are more effective with *any* child, but this is especially true with HSC. It's important to find ways that will help nurture and guide our children rather than break them down.

As parents and caregivers, we need to be mindful of our own reactions and emotions when disciplining. Our children, being their own individual people with unique thoughts and feelings, may not always be happy with the choices or decisions we make for them. Avoiding offensive, defensive, power-loaded, or "giving in" attitudes and, instead, pausing and taking a breath before speaking is a cohesive positive parenting skill that every parent of a highly sensitive child can master through practice and awareness. Watch what happens a couple of times when you stop instead of engaging, and you will see the power of this approach.

You might have seen on parent blogs or magazines that it's best just to let your child cry out their tantrums on their own and ignore the negative behavior in order to teach them it's not okay. However, this approach can send the wrong message, making HSC feel as if they are not heard, seen, understood or accepted. Acknowledging how they feel and allowing them to express their feelings is the key—not offering solutions! Address their reactions with understanding and empathy before discussing solutions, including what is acceptable and what is not. Being there for them both emotionally and physically can create a stronger bond between you, ensuring that they will trust you later on in their most challenging times. And always remember that trust is one of your primary objectives when parenting a highly sensitive child.

When open communication and emotional support are developed, it becomes easier to set boundaries, set limits, and determine how to enforce them. Following through with your disciplinary actions tells your child that they can depend on you and your reaction to their behavior. Provide appropriate consequences, and help your child understand the why behind it for them to learn. Remember, they can only learn when they feel understood and in control. Using open communication that expresses affection, empathy, and confidence in them and your disciplinary action shows them you are on their team and working together.

Most importantly, we need to be aware of our tone when speaking with our HSC. This can be incredibly difficult, especially when we allow ourselves to get frustrated and upset. However, make a conscious effort to keep your tone warm, empathetic, and understanding when talking to your children. We need to provide them with elements of calm and safety by sharing how we are acutely aware of our own emotions, their emotions and the emotions of others. When we do this, they will pick up on our reactions, words, and tones. This supports the overall goal of helping them style their future behaviors, as well.

Parenting a highly sensitive child includes disciplining them, which can be a significant challenge. However, if done correctly, disciplining helps guide them, keeps them on the right path, and models how you work together as a team to get through challenges.

YOUR INTEREST, MY INTEREST

Relationships are just one way children discover who they are and understand those around them. Strong relationships depend on trust and intimacy, and when children experience people helping and understanding them, they find it easier to approach the world with interest and enthusiasm.

When we give them a chance for free play, we allow HSC the autonomy and responsibility of choosing what they'd like to do. Allow your child to take the lead when it comes to playtime and give them your full attention. This will also increase their self-confidence through your confidence and support.

When your child shares with you what they're interested in, respond by focusing your attention on your communication with them. Even if they are showing you something you might not enjoy, such as bugs they found in the yard or video games, be involved in the communication. Show interest and active listening by commenting positively on or describing what they're doing as they do it. This helps your child feel validated, appreciated, and accepted. It also allows you to learn more about them, their interests, and where you have common connections; it establishes authentic trust.

Ask your child to show you how to play their favorite game

or to explain their favorite activity. Even if you already know how, it's a great opportunity to bond as you reverse the roles and allow them to teach you something. This promotes confidence and enthusiasm, and it will give them a sense of pride to be the expert while you act as the learner. Reversing the roles will also teach your child patience as they take on the role of teacher. It will allow them to see things from a new perspective, and you will also be able to see things from their perspective, as well.

Your interest and attention to your child should go beyond playtime. When your child is speaking to you, give them your undivided attention with your ears and body language. HSC will notice small things—even things we aren't consciously doing. When you sense your child wants to talk, face them, and get on their level, look them in the eyes and show that you're really listening. Everyone wants to be heard, especially children.

Pay attention and observe your child for any noticeable behaviors, emotions, or clues in their words or body language. For example, if they are anxiously twisting their fingers together or avoiding eye contact, this gives you valuable information about the level of stress or anxiety they're feeling. It helps to restate what they're saying or make a non-judgmental observation about their emotions to send the message that you're taking them seriously. You could say, "You're telling me you're mad because of this reason, and I can tell it is really upsetting you. Is that correct?" Reflective statements will allow your child to affirm or clarify what they're expressing and can prompt more conversation and understanding.

Whenever they are talking to you, resist the urge to interrupt and correct them while they're speaking. Instead, hear them out and ask follow-up questions to learn more before addressing any problems. This allows you to acknowledge your child's emotions and builds trust between you. They know that you will allow them to speak without interruptions when they come to you. Plus, you're more likely to get better cooperation when you're willing to really pay attention to them rather than immediately correcting them.

Showing an interest in their interests isn't just about showing up or hanging around with them and their activities; it also demonstrates that you are 100% present. By using our body language, communication, and allowing our kids to teach us, we are giving them the respect and appreciation they deserve and modeling how to see the world through other people's perspectives.

DEEP CONNECTION—THE SECRET TO YOUR CHILD'S HEART

Connection is as essential to parents and caregivers as it is to children. It makes parenting easier and more rewarding when we form strong bonds with our kids. Connection helps children want to cooperate if they're able, and it will open up communication lines we might not have otherwise thought possible. When our children trust us to understand them and be their teammates, they're motivated to listen and respect in the same ways we have listened to and respected them.

Research shows that, for every negative interaction, we need at least five positive interactions to help restore a relationship. Since parents spend a lot of time guiding, it's important that this support is positive and that we also invest in doing something besides teaching to maintain this connection with our children. For example, if your child has had a rough day regarding their behavior, try spending a little downtime with them by reading together, playing a game, or watching a movie. Not only will this help calm them, but it will also create a stronger and more positive bond between you.

These are our goals for perfection, but in fact, we're only human, and humans are not perfect. Sometimes all we can do is meet our children's basic needs, and that's all we have to give. It happens. Some days are harder to remain encouraging and supportive. Parenting is one of the hardest jobs in the world. Just do your best with what you have and where you are each moment. Trust in your connection.

Here are ten daily habits of connection you can utilize to keep that bond strong.

1. Share at least 12 physical or emotional connections each day, such as hugs, jokes, special expressions or signals.

Virginia Satir, a family therapist, recommends "four hugs a day for survival, eight for maintenance, and twelve for growth" (Aha! Parenting n.d.). It's always nice to wake up to some snuggles in the morning and to snuggle at night before bedtime. You can also add some physical connections in between by giving pats on the back, tousling the hair, or making eye contact and smiling whenever you can. If physical contact is overwhelming or uncomfortable for your HSC, modify hugs into funny faces or flash cards and embrace the concept of this daily habit for yourself and your child in your own unique way. You'll find that this will also boost your own daily happiness.

2. Play and have fun!

Laughing together and bonding over their interests is a great way to stay connected. It stimulates your child's and your endorphins and oxytocin. Making laughter a priority gives you and your child a chance to laugh off the stress or anxieties you have picked up throughout the day. Playing also encourages children to cooperate.

3. Turn off the technology.

When you're with your child, give them your undivided attention. They will notice if you are preoccupied with your phone, laptop, or TV rather than with them. When you turn off the electronics, you tell your child that they are more important, and they'll remember that when you ask them to turn off *their* electronics and share their full attention with you.

4. Connect with them before transitions.

Change can be hard for children, especially highly sensitive ones. However, when you spend a little time with them one-on-one before a transition, this will help them co-regulate their emotions during these tough times. Look them in the eye, try to get a giggle or smile, and you'll be helping them through the transition in no time.

5. Make time for one-on-one.

If you have just one child, this might be easier. If you have more than one child, spend time with them on their own for at least 10 to 15 minutes a day. Scheduling time individually reinforces how special they are and how much you enjoy and appreciate spending time together.

6. Welcome emotions.

Your highly sensitive child will need to share their feelings with you. This is an opportunity to bring you closer together. Don't let their actions or behaviors trigger your own big feelings. Remain calm and understanding. Acknowledge how they feel and offer understanding rather than advice or criticism. This creates a safe emotional space in which they can come to you about anything and receive empathy and acknowledgment. This will be vital in the future when your highly sensitive child suddenly grows into a highly sensitive teenager. They will need to trust that you will be there without criticism and judgment.

. . .

7. Listen, listen, listen.

Gathering information before trying to interact with your child is super important. It will allow you to gain a better perspective of their point of view and allow your child to be more comfortable sharing with you. It's always polite and respectful to listen to someone without interruption.

8. Slow down.

It's all too easy to get caught up in the rush of our daily schedules. There always seems to be something else that needs to be done or another event to go to. However, try to slow down and savor the moments you have with your child. Whether it's enjoying making breakfast together in the morning or bath time in the evening, give them your full attention and share that moment with love.

9. Bedtime can be a special time.

Your child may already have a routine in order to help go to sleep. However, you might try to set that time a little bit earlier so that you can spend time together winding down. Perhaps you could read them a book before lights-out, or they could read to you. Maybe they can come up with their own stories to tell you from their wild and active imagination. Let this be your special time together. When they're older, late nights may be the only time your teenager might open up to you, so be sure to keep this time sacred and not rush it.

10. Show Up.

If you're a parent with a lot of competing responsibilities, you may not be able to make it to all of your children's activities or special events. However, it's important to at least make the effort. Your children will only be young for a short time, and then—

poof!—they're off on their own. When you are with them, be there 100 percent. Let everything else go and set your worries aside, even if for just a few minutes, to be fully present with your child. Not only will this leave a lasting impression on your child for the rest of their life, but it will give you lasting memories, as well.

We have been gifted with incredible, sensitive, empathetic, intelligent, and amazing children, and we want to encourage and support them as much as possible. Creating a bond with our children will help them explore the world in a secure and confident way and set the tone for their later years. Not only that, but it will help us continue to develop and grow as parents and caregivers.

They won't stay children for long. Make sure they feel just as special as we feel to have them in our lives.

CHAPTER 7

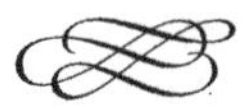

TRAPS TO AVOID IN RAISING THE HIGHLY SENSITIVE CHILD

Highly sensitive children can easily be misunderstood, especially when those closest to them don't understand their temperament. They're often treated as weak despite being incredibly strong when it comes to the number of feelings and stimuli they face daily. Sometimes, it's falsely assumed that they can't handle busy lives or be productive, happy people in general. Being highly sensitive is sometimes mistakenly viewed as a flaw, especially in a society where emotional control and extroversion are considered strengths. Incorrectly judging sensitivity as a weakness or labeling introversion as a problem can inhibit growth and development.

As parents and caregivers, we'd like to think we're above following the social trends and views when it comes to our kids. We believe that we will love them no matter what. Yet, how many times have we caught ourselves thinking about what our child should be doing—whether it's playing a certain sport or being interested in the "right" things. Sometimes, our own perceptions and personal experiences can be so ingrained in our values and belief systems that we aren't even aware we're following them in the first place. This is our opportunity to challenge ourselves to learn, grow, and develop a deeper understanding of how our highly sensitive children function. We can break limiting mindsets in ourselves and be positive models of awareness of the awesome traits of highly sensitive people.

MYTHS ABOUT THE HIGHLY SENSITIVE CHILD/PERSON

The majority of the cultural structures and communication patterns used in today's society were created and reinforced by non-highly sensitive people. This has created several myths about highly sensitive people. Your understanding of these myths will help you become a stronger ambassador for HSP as we create better awareness of this trait in our families and schools and throughout our communities.

Myth #1: Being Highly Sensitive is Not Common

Many people believe that the high sensitivity trait is uncommon when, in actuality, one in five children tend to be more aware of their environment and reactive to stimuli (Gaspari n.d.). HSP have most likely been around throughout our history; however, this trait is only recently being brought to light as research, understanding, and awareness continue to grow.

Myth #2: High Sensitivity is a Mental Disorder

Even as the trait gains more awareness, many people still assume that being highly sensitive is a mental disorder rather than a personality trait. It's fairly common for people unaware of HSP to mislabel a highly sensitive child negatively as being defiant, a crybaby, or socially awkward—or even to misdiagnose them with a mental disorder. However, by now, we know that being highly sensitive isn't a mental disorder, and it doesn't need to be fixed. Instead, with some basic support and understanding, HSC and HSP have a unique perspective and much to offer and share with the world.

Myth #3: Sensitivity is a Weakness

Being highly sensitive is often viewed as a weakness. Many highly sensitive individuals are viewed by people unaware of the trait as unable to handle life's obstacles and challenges. Isn't it beautiful to know that the opposite is generally true? Being highly sensitive means that HSP are handling more than people who are non-HSP and that they are exceptionally strong and capable of doing so. Highly sensitive individuals have different strengths. They're intuitive, imaginative, creative, and compassionate—all things that should be viewed as gifts.

Myth #4: Highly Sensitive People are Incapable of Being Independent

Uninformed people might see occasional outbursts and breakdowns and assume that highly sensitive people can't handle their emotions. In our society, we view an expression of feelings as a sign that a person cannot control themselves. It's almost as if an outward expression of a feeling is an indicator of incompetence. Yet highly sensitive individuals are fully capable of handling their emotions in healthy ways. What's more, their emotional intensity can be an advantage when channeled as passionate energy towards causes they care about. Most people would probably agree that this world benefits from those who clearly understand and express their true emotions and have sincere interest in and deep empathy toward others.

Myth #5: Highly Sensitive People are Shy or Introverted

One of the most often misused labels for highly sensitive individuals is the word "shy." It's common for people unaware of HSP to toss this label around when HSC don't exhibit extroverted traits. The biggest problem with this mislabeling of a highly sensitive child is that it can be self-fulfilling. As a human, if you're repeatedly told you are something, you might actually start to believe it, and your actions will reflect this belief.

Remember, highly sensitive people are not shy; they just tend to observe first before taking action. They prefer making deep, meaningful connections rather than shallow ones with every person they meet, and it usually takes them more time to collect their thoughts before responding. But, like many people, highly sensitive children probably have a lot to say, and they will have no problem saying it when they feel comfortable.

Shyness is a separate behavior from HSP, and it impacts non-highly sensitive and HSP in the same way. The term itself means having a fear of negative judgment in social situations. Highly sensitive people may be incorrectly labeled shy when, in actuality, they are taking a moment to consider all the possibilities of a situation. They reflect and process more than others, which can take more time to get through.

Another label that easily gets misplaced onto a highly sensitive child is "introvert." Because HSC are easily overwhelmed by stimuli and need deep connections to others, highly sensitive individuals may not show outwardly extroverted behaviors. However, this doesn't mean they don't enjoy others' company or that they can't be extroverted. While some highly sensitive people are introverts, other highly sensitive people consider themselves to be extroverted.

Many highly sensitive individuals prefer to have their own space to reflect and recharge; their capacity for authentic, respectful, and sincere relationships makes them natural friends to others. HSP possess caring, loyal, fun, loving, and sincere emotional traits, making them empathetic and compassionate friends.

Myth #6: Highly Sensitive Individuals Cannot Handle Stressful Schedules

Non-highly sensitive people may also falsely believe that highly sensitive individuals cannot thrive with busy lives or excel in specific areas. While self-care is important to everyone, especially those who are highly sensitive, it doesn't always mean taking a break. Highly sensitive people need to be just as careful with under-stimulation as they do over-stimulation. They're happiest when they can put their skills to work in life and relationships, especially if the tasks are highly engaging and creative. They need to find the right intellectual, emotional, and physical stimulation (Weiss 2018).

Myth #7: Highly Sensitive Individuals are Mostly Female

In too many instances, women have been stereotyped as emotional, and society hasn't always allowed men to express their emotions freely. However, men are just as likely to be highly sensitive individuals as women. Dr. Elaine Aron states that this trait is "equally divided between males and females" (Aron n.d.).

Despite this, our social norms tend to deem it more acceptable for women to express their emotions than men. Men often feel the need to be "tough" and suppress their feelings; they're encouraged to hide their sensitive side. Overcoming this social stigma can add significantly to the challenges male HSC and their parents face.

Myth #8: Being Highly Sensitive is Linked to Autism

With the importance and growing awareness about the autism spectrum, another emerging myth is that autism and high sensitivity are related. They are not.

Although people with autism can be highly sensitive, there are also people with an ASD diagnosis who are not highly sensitive. Similarly, there are many people who are highly sensitive and are not autistic. There is no positive relationship between the two, and they should not be conflated.

Myth #9: Being Highly Sensitive is a Bad Thing

Unless people know differently, they may feel that being highly sensitive is a curse rather than a blessing. At times, it can even feel that way to a parent or caregiver—or to the highly sensitive person themself. It's important to remember that this is a genetic trait that comes with profound superpowers. Not only do highly sensitive people have high levels of empathy and the ability to deeply connect with others and with their environment, but there is also a long list of benefits unique to each individual highly sensitive person. Each person brings their own value to the world, and being sensitive doesn't negate that fact.

Myth #10: High Sensitivity Can Be Generalized

It's not uncommon for people to mistake high sensitivity traits for a mental disorder. As with most disorders, highly sensitive people exhibit clear behaviors that make this trait identifiable. Within these identifiable behaviors, each highly sensitive person is unique. No two people are the same, nor do they act exactly the same way. Some HSP are introverts; some are extroverts. Some tend to react to stimuli with outbursts of emotion, while others tend to withdraw. One person might be more sensitive to new environmental situations, while others may be more tuned-in to people's emotions. Temperament traits can be caused by several genes, each with its own small, cumulative effects (Aron n.d.). No two temperaments are the same, so no two highly sensitive children are the same.

There is no right or wrong way to be highly sensitive, and while there are common behaviors, it can be difficult to identify as an outside observer. For example, some highly sensitive individuals may try to suppress their emotions while others express them. In other words, not all highly sensitive people are outwardly emotional. It's always important to understand the individual and not make generalizations about their behaviors.

Myth #11: Being Highly Sensitive is a Choice

Another misconception of high sensitivity is that it's a choice. We now know that high sensitivity is a genetic trait and that it is not a chosen behavior pattern or series of developed habits. Highly sensitive people's nervous systems are wired to this trait—like the color of our hair or eyes.

Myth #12: Highly Sensitive Individuals Struggle with Relationships

Some people—including some HSP—may believe that being highly sensitive is a barrier to forming and maintaining connections. While it is true that HSP often struggle with surface-level interactions, it is simply due to their urge to form deep connections. HSP often get hung up or hurt when it comes to relationships as they expect to find a "perfect" partner. This doesn't mean they struggle with actual relationships any more than anybody else. Relationships are tough for anyone. They require meaningful effort and caring communication, whether a person is highly sensitive or not.

Myth #13: Environments Do Not Affect a Highly Sensitive Child

Interestingly, once people understand that high sensitivity is a temperamental trait, some disregard the child's environment, believing that the child will not change regardless of the environment in which they are raised. However, a highly sensitive child raised in a supportive environment can actually outperform non-sensitive children, academically or socially (Aron n.d.). And

HSC who are raised in negative environments are prone to developing a diagnosis of anxiety or depression. Their environment will affect children no matter their personality or temperament. Supportive and healthy surroundings are important for children to grow and develop into healthy and capable adults, and nothing will change that.

PARENTING TRAPS: STEREOTYPES OF GENDER NORMS

Societal norms promote specific ideas of how men and women dress, behave, and work. These gender roles are based on assigned sex. Women may be expected to dress in what society deems to be more feminine, polite, nurturing, and accommodating. Men may generally be expected to be bold, confident, and exhibit masculine mannerisms. While each community has different gender role expectations, they also change over time.

Gender stereotypes, though over-simplified, lead to unequal and unfair treatment and prejudice and inhibit real personal growth and development. Gender stereotypes are especially harmful for HSP as they do not allow individuals to express themselves or their emotions fully. For example, men may be taught that crying or showing a sensitive emotion is negative, while women may be discouraged from expressing their needs or exhibiting assertive personalities.

Despite the fact that being highly sensitive isn't uncommon, males may not easily admit they're highly sensitive. Our society has encouraged men to be "tough" and has discouraged them from showing their true emotions. Too often, men deny their sensitivities, and they may not even consciously recognize that they are highly sensitive.

When raising a highly sensitive boy, there are some parenting traps to be aware of. Even if you are highly sensitive yourself, raising highly sensitive boys can be exceptionally challenging.

Help them by normalizing their feelings and reminding them that they don't need to hide their emotions to "be tough." As parents and caregivers, we must be careful not to force our children into stereotypical social norms. Forcing them to conform to behaviors that don't align with their natural traits will make highly sensitive boys feel inferior or inadequate. Forcing them to constantly question why they're different rather than embracing their true characteristics undermines their self-awareness, their self-confidence, and the happiness you desire for them.

When we allow our highly sensitive boys to be who they truly are, they will experience an uninhibited life through their unique lens. Being supportive of their sensitivity and nurturing their compassion will lead to great rewards later on.

When it comes to boys, not only are they often not allowed to express emotions openly, but they are too often shamed for outwardly showing fear or displaying a perceived lack of confidence. We need to encourage our highly sensitive boys to experience life while assuring them that failure is not the end of the world or the end of their masculinity. Growth and confidence are not just about mastering something. They are also about knowledge gained from experiences. While you applaud their success, you should focus and encourage their efforts even more than the specific outcome.

Gender roles aren't set in stone, and it's important that we explain this to our children—especially our highly sensitive boys. Teach them that masculinity isn't just about not feeling emotions or vulnerability. Teach and encourage them to be "tough" enough to be confident, kind, compassionate, creative, emotional, and sensitive boys and men. They will thrive with your understanding, respect, and support.

Women and girls are subject to equally harmful generalizations. Too often, women have been dismissed or discriminated against for being highly emotional or sensitive. Girls might be shrugged off simply for being emotional, and their opinions and value are diminished. A recent United Nations report found that nearly 90 percent of men and women globally are biased against females (Conceição et al. 2019). According to this study, close to 50 percent of men surveyed felt they had more rights to a job than women, while nearly half of the men and women globally felt that men made better political leaders. This study also found that there were no countries with true gender equality.

Validate our girls and remind them that while they control their own reactions, they cannot control the actions of others. While they will inevitably learn that there is bias in the world, you can teach them that they are in control of their actions and that they can shape the life they dream about. Help them find healthy ways of managing their reactions and emotions by giving them an outlet for self-care that suits their interests.

Traditional gender roles are rapidly changing, and with our children's strength, as they grow, they will be a part of a future that nurtures sensitivity. Your highly sensitive child's emotions are valid regardless of their gender. Respect your child's feelings by allowing them to open up and, when the time is right, to talk about their perception of gender norms in open, nonjudgmental ways. Never stereotype or ignore your children's emotions, and always honor them for their feelings and the insights and value that they bring to a situation and to their relationships.

PARENTS, DON'T LISTEN TO THIS!

When it comes to parenting in general, people love to share their own opinions on how you should raise your child. There are countless parenting books, theories, and styles to learn from. There always seems to be a friendly neighbor or fellow parent who thinks of themself as an expert on children after having one themself. However, there are harmful parenting tips and advice out there to be aware of.

High sensitivity is a trait that is too often critically judged, and because both strangers and loved ones enjoy giving unsolicited advice about parenting, you've probably heard some of the negative comments below. If you hear these, pay no mind to them.

1. "They'll need to get thicker skin."

Research says otherwise. Highly sensitive children are wired differently; it's not just a case of having "thin skin." They show higher levels of empathy, awareness, and processing. It's unlikely this will ever change. While HSC can find ways to regulate and manage their emotional reactions, they will always be their sensitive selves. We should embrace that quality within them rather than trying to toughen it out.

2. "They're really emotional."

Even if this is an accurate observation, it's not helpful if presented in a judgemental or condescending way. If someone says this to you, let them know that, yes, your child is sensitive and why it's a positive attribute. Take time to share with them that your child is deeply processing their surroundings and emotions and that their awareness is a gift.

3. "They're manipulating you."

Children are not natural-born schemers. When they show emotion, it is their way of communicating how they feel when they're unable to put their emotions into words. Highly sensitive children have an exceptionally lower threshold for stimulation and express strong emotions. Don't take it personally. It is not meant to be manipulative; it's a means of communication.

4. "Sometimes we just have to force kids to do the things they don't want to do."

While this can certainly apply to safety measures such as

holding your hand out on the street, it does not apply to social situations. When children are uncomfortable in a situation, we should respect them. They will have plenty of time to learn what they can handle and what they cannot without forcing it on them when they're not ready. When they are confident enough and able to handle a new experience, they'll conquer it—but we need to give them that safety and stability first.

5. "You need to let them grow up at some point."

Listening to your child's needs doesn't make you an overprotective or coddling parent. You know when your child is ready to face a challenge or new experience better than anyone else. You also know when your child needs some extra time to warm up to new people or situations. Allowing our children to grow at their own pace is a positive parenting approach and a gift to both of you. There's no need to put pressure on your child to become self-reliant before they're ready. With guidance and support, they will eventually get there.

WRONG LABELING

Even after learning what it means to be a highly sensitive individual, HSP and HSC might be hesitant to talk about this trait with others. Being sensitive is often societally regarded as a weakness, which we might understand to be ridiculous—but outside judgment is often very real. It is common for people unaware of what high sensitivity really is, including teachers, parents, and caregivers, to mislabel HSC as shy or offer a misguided "armchair diagnosis" of an unrelated mental health disorder.

Francesca Lionetti, a researcher at Queen Mary University of London, used a popular metaphor to define childhood behavioral patterns. She states that children fall into three groups: orchids, who are highly sensitive and need particular environments to thrive; dandelions, who can grow virtually anywhere; and tulips, who fall in between these two extremes (Lionetti et al. 2018). Highly sensitive children flourish with the right support. For our orchids, the understanding and support of the teachers, parents, and caregivers around them play a vital role in their development.

Studies have found links between extreme psychobiological reactivity and predisposed temperament characteristics, such as shyness or the need to avoid new situations (Boyce 2020). For orchids, their defining feature is their sensitivity to social situations, and, as such, their environment impacts them more than dandelions or tulips. While it's true that any child thrives in a protective, positive, and loving environment, orchids positively bloom.

Even the most well-intentioned but uninformed educators are sometimes confused when they learn how stressful it is for these types of students to be boxed into a standard school-based setting. Instead of forcing HSC to conform to the social norms that schools often reinforce, we need to help their teachers understand their needs. For example, if they get anxious in the classroom, recognize that they may need to take a few minutes to find a quiet place to breathe, take a walk, or collect themselves while they calm down.

When you hear inappropriate statements or wrong labels, you can do your best to help teach people what it really means to be highly sensitive. But, above all else, the best way to combat any negative labeling is to make sure your child knows just how special and amazing they are. Words can hurt, but when you give your highly sensitive child the love and support they need, they can handle anything thrown their way.

THE TRAP OF EMOTIONAL NEGLECT

Emotional neglect is defined as a "relationship pattern in which an individual's affectional needs are consistently disregarded, ignored, invalidated, or unappreciated" (Levine, Carey, and

Crocker 1992). When a child's emotional and developmental needs are not met, it leads to immediate and long-term consequences. Emotional neglect is not necessarily emotional abuse; the latter comes from intentional mistreatment, while emotional neglect is a failure to notice or act on a child's needs. Parents may provide basic care and necessities to their children while still emotionally neglecting them.

Brushing off or disregarding our children's emotions is just one way we can emotionally neglect them. When our child tells us their feelings about something we believe to be of little consequence, we're invalidating their emotions and ignoring their needs. The effects of this can be subtle, and many parents may not realize they're even doing it. It's also difficult for other caregivers and educators to recognize the small but neglectfully hurtful actions that especially impact an HSC. Understanding the behaviors and actions of emotional neglect are vital for parents and caregivers as we nurture the growth of our HSC.

The most common symptoms of emotional neglect can be obvious, but be aware of subtle ones, as well; they might not show up immediately. If the neglect continues, symptoms and consequences become more serious over time. Symptoms can include depression, anxiety, apathy, hyperactivity, aggression, developmental delays, low self-esteem, substance misuse, withdrawal, indifference, or shunning emotional intimacy (Holland and Legg 2021).

Those who struggle with emotional neglect as children can grow into adults with lasting consequences of their childhood neglect. Neglect as a child has been linked to an increased risk of developing mental disorders such as anxiety or depression. A study conducted by Glickman et al. found that higher levels of emotional neglect were linked to increased depressive symptoms at the age of 18 (2021). Although most children who have experienced neglect do not neglect their own children when they become parents themselves, research suggests that they are at a higher risk of neglecting their children, compared to parents who were not neglected in their childhood (Yang et al. 2018).

I'd like to note that if you read this and feel like you may have emotionally neglected your child, please, give yourself some grace. This book is about love, awareness, and positive solutions as we understand how to care for our HSC and our relationships with them. Now that you are aware, you can make a mindful effort to help create an emotionally supportive environment. If you are concerned that your child is experiencing anxiety, depression, or symptoms of emotional neglect, you can provide them with additional support with a qualified therapist or practitioner. Remember to address your own needs, as well; "put on your own mask before helping others" is a valid metaphor for parenting. Finding ways to understand and support yourself is the only way you can effectively support your child in *their* life journey.

Supportive clinical therapy can be extremely beneficial. Having a competent therapist to talk with can help both you and your child when you're struggling. Seeking professional help is commendable, and there are often significant benefits to it.

Emotional neglect can damage a child's mental health and confidence. It teaches them that their feelings are not important. These consequences can manifest themselves over a lifetime if not resolved. As I've stated a few times throughout this book, it's vital for us as parents and caregivers to acknowledge, accept, and encourage our highly sensitive child's emotions. Finding your own superpower and support is critical for both of you. Explore and practice the extra efforts needed to make sure they understand just how loved, understood, and valuable they are.

MAKING THEM FEEL WANTED

All children want to feel wanted. They need to feel loved. This may seem obvious, but there are subtle things we can easily miss when it comes to our highly sensitive children. Expressed love is the key principle in helping your child grow stronger. It's just as important as food, shelter, or water and builds a child's foundation of competency and resiliency. It helps improve their overall mental wellness and can even make them physically healthier. Love and affection boost your child's brain development and create a stronger connection between you, helping your child avoid the consequences of emotional neglect.

One way we can help show our love to our children is by waking them up in a positive way. Studies have shown there are nine minutes during the day that have the biggest influence on children: the first three minutes after waking up, three minutes after they come home from school or an activity, and the last three minutes before they go to sleep (Wiatrak 2019).

Think about how you wake up. Do you have a better day when you wake up in a positive way, such as with a gentle touch, a shared smile, a welcoming scene out the window, or a comfortable and inviting environment? Children are no different. Think of what might be best for your child to wake up to. Maybe it's playing their favorite song in the morning and dancing along with you as you get ready. Or maybe it's preparing a favorite breakfast. Whatever it might be, do it! You will be teaching your child how to set a positive tone for their day and helping them build a routine for waking up and starting the day feeling refreshed and happy.

As I've mentioned before, when sharing one-on-one time with your child, be sure to look and listen to whatever it is that they are doing or saying. When you give them your undivided attention, this makes them feel valued and wanted. Truly engage with your child by asking questions and being fully present. Take your child out for special "date nights" or do a special activity at home.

Creating fun and new traditions can make your child feel extra special. Perhaps you can make plans to go to the library on a specific day of the week or take your children out for an "ice cream night" once a month. Making a tradition specifically for them is just one way you can show your special love.

BECOMING OVERPROTECTIVE

All parents want to protect their children. It's something that's been programmed into us for centuries. Our children depend on us to offer them safety and love. However, we need to learn when it's time to protect and when it's time to let our children learn on their own.

Hovering too close and trying to keep them in a protective bubble can do more harm than good. Children learn through experiences, and they cannot learn if you do not give them chances to have their own experiences. Finding that sweet spot in keeping your children safe while not being overprotective is mostly trial and error, but you must keep trying.

Here are some ways to help you empower your children and guide them towards independence.

First, there is a difference between risk and risky behaviors. Take, for example, teaching your child to ride a bike. There is a risk they will fall, but through that experience, they learn to balance. However, riding their bike along the highway—now, *that's* risky. When you help your child to understand the difference between risk and risky behaviors, they'll soon be able to make their own decisions about what is a reasonable risk and what is dangerous, risky business.

You can help your child understand risks by practicing safety. Show and assist them with properly using their bike, playground equipment, or anything else they'd like to try before letting them do it on their own. This way, you'll be giving them the tools they will need to do it independently while still being aware of safety.

Not only will this help keep them safe, but you'll be providing them with the necessary life skills they will need later on. Allowing your kids to grow their sense of independence will teach them competence and boost their confidence as they learn what they're capable of without the help of their parents.

If something feels unsafe, it's okay to tell your children why you're worried. Show them how you deal with those concerns in a healthy way by addressing safety. When children see you worrying, they learn through that model how to deal with their own fears in life. Remind yourself that you are teaching your child how to be safe, resilient, and, ultimately, independent. HSC are hyper-aware of our emotions and feelings; your stress will only make them more anxious.

If you identify as a parent with helicopter tendencies who is hoping to be more relaxed, try avoiding spending time with other parents who are also overprotective. Their anxiety and fears might be rubbing off on you without you even realizing it. Plus, watching them swoop in to rescue their children every second might make you relapse to your old ways. Instead, surround yourself with parents and caregivers who are solid examples of allowing their children the freedom you want for your child. This will reinforce what you feel to be right and help support your decision to give your child more autonomy and independence.

It's natural to feel protective of your children. You know your limits and your child's limits better than anyone else. However, stifling their freedom and creativity to take risks can be detrimental to their growth and learning. By teaching them safety and problem-solving skills and helping them understand risky behavior, we give them the necessary guidelines and tools they need to find their own autonomy.

CHAPTER 8

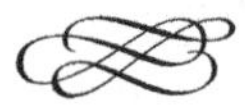

GUIDING THEM THROUGH AND THROUGH

Being a parent of a highly sensitive child is an intense responsibility and a great privilege. It's an honor to witness their incredible capacities for intuition, insight, observation, compassion, and love. It's a responsibility because they are easily hurt and struggle to channel their strong emotions. It is a privilege because being a part of their journey and providing the guidance and supportive environment they need gives you a front-row seat as you watch them thrive as positive, resilient, productive, passionate, and happy individuals.

Here are a few more exercises you can add to your parenting toolbox to help encourage your highly sensitive children's confidence, compassion, calmness, and resilience.

YOU CAN DO THIS—YOUR RADICAL CONFIDENCE

Dear parents and caregivers of highly sensitive children:

Parenting comes with a lot of self-doubts for every parent. Are you giving them enough independence? Are you meeting their physical and emotional needs? Are you doing enough in general? The worries and self-doubt can feel endless.

Take a deep breath and give yourself some space and grace.

Celebrate your accomplishments. Remind yourself again that there is nothing "wrong" with you or your highly sensitive child. Go deep! You need to really and truly believe this. You are clearly doing your best to give your highly sensitive child the love and support they need. Although you may be the best person to help your child grow and achieve their dreams, you do not have to do it all alone. You may find that you can best help your child by coordinating others to help assist in many different areas. I like to think of this strategy as being the conductor, rather than a solo musician, in the symphony of your child's life. Learning to delegate roles and activities to others is not a weakness; it expands your child's network and experiences of support and understanding.

Remember, your child's sensitivity—and everything that comes with it—is a gift. Sure, it comes with its unique challenges, but no matter what, you're going to be there for them. As long as you keep believing that your child is special, beautiful, and amazing, they will, too.

You have the power to help your child have the confidence and self-esteem they need to navigate life's obstacles. You're the compass to help your child find their direction and the map to help them plot their own course for their life.

Whether it is you directly or your guidance in coordinating with others for your children, your core principles are always:

- Keep loving your child, just as they are.
- Let them be free to express themselves and help them when they cannot.
- Give them a voice and a platform to be heard.
- Show them that they matter.

When you do these things, you will have the reward of witnessing them conquer whatever challenges come between them and their goals.

Believe in yourself and your abilities; listen to your intuition.

Everyone has an opinion on how you should raise your child, but you know best. Trust yourself and, when you feel doubt, seek self-care and calmly find ways to grow your understanding for ways to share love with your child.

Just as your highly sensitive child is learning how to adjust to this world, you are also learning about yourself and how to parent them in ways that work for both of you. This book is a stepping stone to laying down a path of understanding. You are on exactly the right path, so just keep going!

TEACHING THEM TO APPRECIATE THE UNIQUENESS IN OTHERS

Although HSC are usually more empathetic and compassionate toward others, they're still kids, and even though most parents want to raise kind and caring children, that priority can get lost when stacked up against academics, activities, or social pressures. It's nice to think that most parents encourage kindness in their kids—ourselves included. However, according to the study "Making Caring Common" by Harvard psychologist Richard Weissbourd, that's not the case.

His study found approximately 80 percent of children have reported that their parents are more concerned with their own achievement or happiness compared to exhibiting care for other people (Joyce 2021). The children also were three times more likely to agree that their parents were more proud of their academic success than the act of being a caring community member.

According to the Making Caring Common study, there are five strategies to help raise caring children (Joyce 2021).

1. Make caring for others a priority in your household.

Parents tend to prioritize how their child is treated more than how their child treats others—and that's perfectly normal. But children need to find a balance between their own needs and the needs of others. They can learn from you that caring for other people is a priority and the best way to do this is by holding them accountable to those expectations. For example, before your child quits an activity, ask them to consider what commitment they made to other people when they first joined and how it might affect those other people if they choose to leave. One of the best ways is to model the behavior you want to see in your own children by being kind and respectful to others. Open communication about healthy boundaries is useful if you see them falling into the trappings of "people-pleasing" behaviors. Your sincere conversations and authentic examples are natural tools for teaching your children.

2. Provide learning opportunities for your child to practice being kind.

Children learn by watching and doing. Learning to care for others is just like learning any other skill. You can encourage them to help a friend with homework, chip in around the house, and find other opportunities to practice helping people. Try not to reward your child for being helpful when it's expected, such as with basic chores, but definitely reward them for acts of kindness that you don't expect, such as helping someone they see struggling in a social situation.

3. Expand your child's circle of concern.

Most of the time, your children naturally care about their close family and friends. But what about those outside of their usual circle? Helping them be aware of how their actions affect others in public areas and around people they aren't close to allows them to understand their impact on the world. Take every opportunity to broaden their exposure and experiences with the big picture of the world around them by teaching them about people who live in different cultures or communities outside of their own. Show your HSC that they are a valuable part of this world filled with interesting people, places, and opportunities.

4. Model how to care for others.

As parents, we are our HSC's biggest role models, and, as such, we should show them how it's done. When we care about others, our children will pick up on that. When we practice honesty, fairness, and caring, we show our children a positive model for how to live their lives. If you have the time, you may even want to find a local cause for which you and your child can volunteer together.

5. Help your child deal with their negative feelings in a healthy way.

Sometimes, our ability to care for others can be overpowered by anger, shame, envy, or other feelings. As we teach our HSC that feeling these emotions is okay and normal, we also need to teach them the difference between helpful and unhelpful ways to deal with them. Hopefully, some of the ideas in this book are already helping you.

DAILY EXERCISES IN SELF-ACCEPTANCE AND COMPASSION

Most people agree that the world benefits from kindness and empathy. Imagine what our world would be like if every single home around the globe encouraged kindness and compassion during their child's developmental years. And while it's important to improve our community, did you know that nurturing kindness and empathy can also help improve emotional intelligence?

There are lots of strategies to teach kindness. Some you've already read above. Here are a few more examples of daily exercises you may choose to add to your routine to help encourage self-acceptance and compassion.

Starting a family "kindness jar" is a simple positive reinforcement system that can help encourage kind behavior. This is a jar that your children can decorate, which makes it extra fun, especially for HSC who are creative. At the beginning of each day, have your child write one kindness note by filling in this sentence; "I am kind when I…." Then, place it into the kindness jar. At the end of the day, have your children read their notes and ask if they were able to be kind today. Allow them to tell you about their act of kindness that day and reflect on how they treated others at school or a social event.

Books about friendship provide valuable learning and discussion time. Have your child pick out a book with a kindness theme and read it together. At the end of the book, try to engage your child by asking questions about what they could or would do in those hypothetical situations.

Each day, you can also take a little time to act out scenarios in which your child will choose to respond with compassion. This could happen during playtime, or you could carve out a special time to do this with your child. Treat it as role-playing and make it fun. Some examples of scenarios you can act out with your child are:

- Noticing someone who is alone who seems sad.
- Someone fell down and hurt themselves.
- Their sibling is sick (or parent if they are an only child).
- Their parent just came home from work, and it's been an exhausting day.
- They notice a person who is disabled struggling to open a door.
- Someone in their class had a pet who passed away and is very sad about it.

You can use these scenarios or make up your own. Whatever you choose to do, role-playing different situations with your child can help them practice being kind. Eventually, it will be second nature to them, and they will grow to be caring and compassionate adults.

If your child is old enough to write, you can help them start a "Gratitude Journal." Have them write down, or talk about, one to three things they're grateful for each day. This could be done in their downtime when they need to recharge, as it gives them a quiet space to reflect on their day and relax. By writing down what they're grateful for, they will start noticing more positive things in their lives and practice optimism. This will also encourage them to be kinder towards others as they will be more aware that they might have something others don't. If you'd like to read more about how to cultivate a positive practice, you can check out my daily journals or my book, *The Guide to Gratitude: Cultivate Your Positivity Practice for a Life Filled with Happiness, Mindfulness, and Thankfulness*, available on Amazon.

These daily activities don't take long to complete and can easily be implemented into your usual daily routine. Your child will be practicing being kind to others and will be able to reflect on their own actions in real-life scenarios.

CALMNESS EXERCISES

Highly sensitive children need to learn how to calm themselves when feeling overwhelmed by their environment or emotions. Here are a few suggestions that may help you calm your highly sensitive child and allow them to learn to manage and regulate their feelings in a healthy way. Things such as drinking water, visualizing a quiet place, or channeling their energy into exercise or creative activities can help them find their happy place until they are calm once more.

When you've had a long day at work, a nice hot bath can be the perfect thing right when you get home. The same may be true for your HSC. Using bath time may help children wind down after an exhausting or exciting day. If you're finding that your child is having a bad day in general, you may want to set up the bathroom to be as relaxing as possible and let your child chill out until they're feeling better.

If your child needs a distraction from their negative emotions during the day, try practicing a mantra they can use when they're feeling stressed or overwhelmed. It can be something simple such as "I am calm" or "I am relaxed." Make it easy to remember and practice it with them. Eventually, they will use this technique to self-regulate their emotions.

For older children, keeping a journal can be extremely therapeutic and help them process difficult emotions. Writing their feelings can have a profound effect on their mental health and mood. Allow them to write how they truly feel and resist the urge to read it. You want your child to trust you, which may mean giving them an outlet to explore how they feel private from your eyes.

You can use stress balls or other fidget toys to help calm HSC down. While fidget spinners can sometimes be misused and turned into a distraction, especially in the classroom, they can also be extremely helpful for the children who really need them for comfort or self-care. Keep in mind that a technique may be appropriate in different situations or at different times.

Remind your child that it is okay to walk away from stressful situations when they need a break. This might be the hardest thing to do, but you can help them by practicing this together. Sometimes, children need a change of scenery to calm down. Whether it's just walking into another room or taking a walk outside, this change can reset their emotional state.

These are just a few calming ideas and techniques your child can learn to do on their own. When your child is able to control their emotions and calm down, it can help them face their problems with a clear head and find their own solutions.

NURTURE YOURSELF TOO

One of our biggest goals as parents of highly sensitive children is to be patient. That's a lot easier said than done. To be calm and composed, we need to be able to nurture ourselves, just as we nurture our HSC.

Self-care isn't just key to remaining patient; it also helps us relax, and when we're relaxed, so are our children. If you find yourself feeling exhausted or depleted or your patience is running thin, it may be time to take a self-care day—or two.

Pay attention to what your body is telling you. If you're feeling overwhelmed or stressed, try taking in deep breaths. Close your eyes and listen to your body as you breathe. Sometimes, taking a break for yourself is what your body and mind need.

Consciously parent yourself. Nurture your inner child. Talk to yourself in a loving, caring way and acknowledge your efforts, successes, and mistakes. Understand that you're not perfect, nor do you need to be. Be kind to yourself.

It's especially important to take care of your mental health while parenting and caring for your HSC. If you're not feeling your best, your highly sensitive child will notice that and possibly reflect it—it may rub off on them. I hear parents say that they are willing to die for their kids, but my question is, are they willing to *live* for them? Practice the self-care you need and show them how to live a healthy life.

FINAL WORDS

Parenting is never an easy job, and raising a highly sensitive child comes with even more twists and challenges—but here you are, trying to understand the incredible world of your highly sensitive child. You are collecting the necessary tools to help support and guide you and your child throughout life. It's my sincere hope that you have found this book helpful.

Although raising a highly sensitive child can be overwhelming at times, you are becoming a stronger parent. The key to your success is to stay calm and have a plan for when your HSC shows signs of distress. Demonstrate empathy and help guide them—model how you personally manage challenges and stress and teach them techniques to regulate their emotions and feelings. The more you work on this, the easier it gets.

Remember that being highly sensitive is not a disorder but a personality trait—that highly sensitive children are neuro-diverse and experience intensely vivid sensory stimuli.

Throughout this book, we have emphasized that validating their emotions and providing empathetic support and understanding are crucial to helping your highly sensitive child. The environment you create for them and the behaviors you model are critically important for their development. Our orchids can blossom when we provide routines, calming techniques, downtime, and safe spaces for them to grow. In order to do this, understand their personality, triggers, and emotional tendencies to know which tactics you need to use in particular situations and at particular times.

Encourage your HSC in their already empathetic and compassionate natures, and when things get a bit rough, show them how to deal with high waves and tough currents. In this book, we've listed a few helpful techniques for you and your child, such as breathing exercises, practicing gratitude, and using positive affirmations to help build their self-confidence.

Highly sensitive children need support, love, understanding, and empathy. You're there for many of their steps along the way to make sure that they really understand just how special they are and that their emotions are valid.

You are learning that it's not only your child you are striving to understand but also yourself. Take a look at how you behave each day and how you react to stress and unexpected change. You can model the behavior and stress-coping mechanisms you want your child to learn. Always remember that you are not alone and that you can access support for yourself and your child. Whether you are a highly sensitive parent or not, parenting HSC sometimes feels like a daunting task. Please be gentle as you remember this: we're all human. We all make mistakes. We all have our highs and our lows. With the right love, respect, and support, our highly sensitive children will blossom and grow beyond our wildest imaginations! You and your HSC are not "normal;" you and your HSC are uniquely yourselves.

You're already doing great! And after adapting some of these ideas from this book to fit into your life, you'll do even better. You now have the tools you need to get out there and do your best. You have the enhanced understanding and competence to keep doing your best. You have expanded knowledge and insights that will help you along this journey. Congratulations on being an exceptional parent for an exceptional child.

REFERENCES

Aha! Parenting. "10 Habits to Strengthen Your Relationship with Your Child." AhaParenting.com. Accessed January 31, 2022. https://www.a-haparenting.com/read/10-habits-to-stay-connected-to-your-child.

APA Dictionary of Psychology, s.v. "inferiority complex." Accessed January 31, 2022. https://dictionary.apa.org/inferiority-complex.

Aron, Elaine. "FAQ: How Do I Know For Sure That I Am Highly Sensitive Or That MyChild Is Highly Sensitive?" The Highly Sensitive Person. Accessed January 31, 2022. https://hsperson.com/faq/how-do-i-know-for-sure/.

Betancort, Moisés. "The Highly Sensitive Brain." E-motion: Potential of Highlysensitivity, April 6, 2020. https://highlysensitive.eu/en/the-highly-sensitive-brain/.

Boyce, W. Thomas. *The Orchid and the Dandelion: Why Some Children Struggle and How All Can Thrive.* London: Bluebird, 2020. ISBN-10: 1509805176.

Cascio, Christopher N., Matthew Brook O'Donnell, Francis J. Tinney, Matthew D. Lieberman, Shelley E. Taylor, Victor J. Strecher, and Emily B. Falk. "Self-Affirmation Activates Brain Systems Associated with Self-Related Processing and Reward and Is Reinforced by Future Orientation." *Social Cognitive and Affective Neuroscience* 11, no. 4 (2015): 621–29. https://doi.org/10.1093/scan/nsv136.

Child Trends. "Databank Indicator Archive." Accessed January 31, 2022. https://www.childtrends.org/indicators?a-z.

Conceição, Pedro, Jon Hall, Yu-Chieh Hsu, Admir Jahic, Milorad Kovacevic, Tanni Mukhopadhyay, Anna Ortubia, Carolina Rivera, and Heriberto Tapia. "Tackling Social Norms: A Game Changer For Gender Inequalities." UNDP 2020 Human Development Perspectives, 2020. http://hdr.undp.org/sites/default/files/hd_perspectives_gsni.pdf.

Daw, Jonathan, Michael Shanahan, Kathleen Mullan Harris, Andrew Smolen, Brett Haberstick, and Jason D. Boardman. "Genetic Sensitivity to Peer Behaviors." *Journal of Health and Social Behavior* 54, no. 1 (2013): 92–108. https://doi.org/10.1177/0022146512468591.

Drudi, Cassandra. "9 Signs You Have a Highly Sensitive Kid." Today's Parent, August 12, 2021. https://www.todaysparent.com/kids/kids-health/signs-you-have-a-highly-sensitive-child/amp/.

Eby, Douglas. "Shyness, Introversion, Sensitivity – What's the Difference?" Highly Sensitive, December 13, 2021. https://highlysensitive.org/11343/shyness-introversion-sensitivity-whats-the-difference/.

Fernandez, Sonia. "Scans Peek at Brains of Highly Sensitive People." Futurity, May 6, 2021. https://www.futurity.org/highly-sensitive-people-brains-2559912-2/.

Gaspari, Maureen. "5 Myths About The Highly Sensitive Child." The Highly Sensitive Child Accessed January 31, 2022. https://www.thehighlysensitivechild.com/5-myths-about-the-highly-sensitive-child/.

Gere, Douglas R., Steve C. Capps, D. Wayne Mitchell, and Erin Grubbs. "Sensory Sensitivities of Gifted Children." *The American Journal of Occupational Therapy* 63, no. 3 (2009): 288–95. https://doi.org/10.5014/ajot.63.3.288.

Glickman, Emma A., Karmel W. Choi, Alexandre A. Lussier, Brooke J. Smith, and Erin C. Dunn. "Childhood Emotional Neglect and Adolescent Depression: Assessing the Protective Role of Peer Social Support in a Longitudinal Birth Cohort." *Frontiers in Psychiatry* 12 (2021). https://doi.org/10.3389/fpsyt.2021.681176.

Goleman, Daniel. *Emotional Intelligence: The 25th Anniversary Edition*. New York: Bantam Books, 2020. ISBN-10: 1526633620.

Highly Sensitive Society. "Highly Sensitive Person." Accessed January 31, 2022. https://www.highlysensitivesociety.com/highlysensitiveperson.

Holland, Kimberly, and Timothy J. Legg. "Childhood Emotional Neglect: What It Is, and How It Can Affect You." Healthline, October 21, 2021. https://www.healthline.com/health/mental-health/childhood-emotional-neglect#symptoms-in-children.

Jagiellowicz, Jadzia. "HSP And Sensory Processing Disorder." Highly Sensitive Society, November 20, 2019. https://www.highlysensitivesociety.com/blog/hspandsensoryprocessingdisorder.

Joyce, Amy. "Are You Raising Nice Kids? A Harvard Psychologist Gives 5 Ways to Raise Them to Be Kind." *The Washington Post*, October 24, 2021. https://www.washingtonpost.com/news/parenting/wp/2014/07/18/are-you-raising-nice-kids-a-harvard-psychologist-gives-5-ways-to-raise-them-to-be-kind/?outputType=amp.

Lear, Katie. "Is Your Child A Highly Sensitive Person?" Child Counseling In Davidson, January 7, 2021. https://www.katielear.com/child-therapy-blog/2020/10/26/highly-sensitive-child-symptoms.

Lionetti, Francesca, Arthur Aron, Elaine N. Aron, G. Leonard Burns, Jadzia Jagiellowicz, and Michael Pluess. "Dandelions, Tulips and Orchids: Evidence for the Existence of Low-Sensitive, Medium-Sensitive and High-Sensitive Individuals." *Translational Psychiatry* 8, no. 1 (2018). https://doi.org/10.1038/s41398-017-0090-6.

Lodestone Center for Behavioral Health. "Highly Sensitive Children." Accessed January 31, 2022. https://www.lodestonecenter.com/highly-sensitive-children/.

NIMH. "Mental Illness." National Institute of Mental Health. Accessed January 31, 2022. https://www.nimh.nih.gov/health/statistics/mental-illness.

Schiffman, Richard. "Is Your Child an Orchid, a Tulip or a Dandelion?" *The New York Times*, August 6, 2020. https://www.nytimes.com/2020/08/06/well/family/sensitive-child.html.

Smolewska, Kathy A., Scott B. McCabe, and Erik Z. Woody. "A Psychometric Evaluation of the Highly Sensitive Person Scale: The Components of Sensory-Processing Sensitivity and Their Relation to the BIS/Bas and 'Big Five.'" *Personality and Individual Differences* 40, no. 6 (2006): 1269–79. https://doi.org/10.1016/j.paid.2005.09.022.

Yang, Mi-Youn, Sarah A. Font, McKenzie Ketchum, and Youn Kyoung Kim. "Intergenerational Transmission of Child Abuse and Neglect: Effects of Maltreatment Type and Depressive Symptoms." *Children and Youth Services Review* 91 (2018): 364–71. https://doi.org/10.1016/j.childyouth.2018.06.036.

Wiatrak, Brandi. "20 Ways To Make Your Child Feel Loved And

Valued." The Cultured Baby, June 14, 2019. https://theculturedbaby.-world/2019/06/14/ways-to-make-your-child-feel-loved-and-valued/amp/.

Weiss, Suzannah. "7 Myths To Stop Believing About Highly Sensitive People." Bustle, July 18, 2018. https://www.bustle.com/p/7-myths-to-stop-believing-about-highly-sensitive-people-9752736.

Wilson, Catherine. "Checklist Of Traits In Highly Sensitive Children." Focus On The Family. Accessed January 31, 2022. https://www.focusonthefamily.ca/content/checklist-of-traits-in-highly-sensitive-children.

Special Request

Could you please do me a favor? If you enjoyed this book and found it helpful, would you be so kind as to review on Amazon? Reviews are extremely important for any future reader looking for more positive parenting solutions to raise highly sensitive children. If you see the value of sharing these concepts with others, please take two minutes to leave a review.

To demonstrate my appreciation for your review and feedback, email me at jon@exploringchanges.com with a link to your verified review and receive a free 60-minute coaching session. If it's a good fit, you will also qualify to receive a 20% discount on any coaching package.

THANK YOU, THANK YOU, THANK YOU SO MUCH!

Other Books by Jonathan Baurer:

The Guide to Gratitude:

Cultivate Your Positivity Practice for a Life Filled with Happiness, Mindfulness and Thankfulness 21 Daily Journal Exercises

Scan this QR code to purchase

Made in the USA
Coppell, TX
19 December 2022